*An Introduction to the
General P   ogy of T*

An Introduction to the General Pathology of Tumours

By David J. B. Ashley T.D., M.D., F.R.C.PATH.
Consultant Pathologist, Morriston Hospital, Swansea

Bristol: John Wright & Sons Ltd 1972

COPYRIGHT NOTICE

© D. J. B. Ashley, 1972

All Rights Reserved. No part of this publication may be reproduced, stored in a retrieval system, or transmitted, in any form or by any means, electronic, mechanical, photocopying, recording, or otherwise, without the prior permission of John Wright & Sons Ltd.

Distribution by Sole Agents:
United States of America: The Williams & Wilkins Company, Baltimore
Canada: The Macmillan Company of Canada Ltd., Toronto

ISBN 0 7236 0319 7

PRINTED IN GREAT BRITAIN BY JOHN WRIGHT & SONS LTD.,
AT THE STONEBRIDGE PRESS, BRISTOL BS4 5NU

PREFACE

THIS small book is offered as a contribution to the application of general medical and scientific principles to the understanding of neoplastic disease in the human. It is directed to the clinician, both undergraduate and postgraduate, who is concerned with the care and management of patients suffering from neoplastic disease and who wants a résumé of current knowledge in this field. The emphasis is on neoplastic disease in humans and the tone is necessarily didactic. Detailed pro and con arguments are not generally presented and the evidence used is not justified in detail. Such expositions are available in larger works intended for a somewhat different group of readers.

It should be emphasized that the field of tumour pathology is not static. Fresh knowledge, fresh concepts, and fresh correlations are continuously appearing, both from workers in this discipline and also from other fundamental, applied, and clinical studies. An essential mode of thought of the worker in Scientific Medicine is that he must be prepared to accept change and new ideas from any direction. I hope that this work may be useful as a peninsula from which to proceed towards a fuller understanding.

I am indebted for the ideas presented here to a vast army of colleagues who have stimulated my thoughts by their writings, by their sayings, and by their discussions and questions. I trust that, in turn, I may be able to help others to face, in their daily practice, one of the common lethal disorders of mankind.

Four of my colleagues, Dr. E. A. Danino, Dr. R. W. Evans, Mr. J. E. Mitchell, and Mr. G. L. Williams, have helped me by criticizing the manuscript. I am most grateful to them for their assistance.

I am also most grateful to my research assistant, Mrs. Molly Rees, B.A., who has typed and retyped the manuscript and has never lost patience with the vagaries of the author.

D. J. B. A.

Swansea, September 1971

CONTENTS

Chapter	Page
Preface	v
I.—Introduction	1
II.—Definitions and Classification	3
III.—Clinicopathological Correlation in Tumours	11
IV.—The Spread of Tumours	19
V.—Differentiation, Dedifferentiation, and Tumour Histology	25
VI.—The Precancerous State: Carcinoma-in-situ	32
VII.—Progression and Regression	38
VIII.—Oncogenesis	43
IX.—Genetics and Tumours	47
X.—Environmental Factors in Tumour Formation	55
XI.—Viruses and Tumours	65
XII.—Hormones and Tumours	73
XIII.—Immunity and Tumours	85
XIV.—The Pathological Basis of the Chemotherapy of Tumours	92
XV.—Teratomata	98
Further Reading	102
Index	103

An Introduction to the General Pathology of Tumours

CHAPTER I

INTRODUCTION

IN the present-day practice of Medicine in the developed countries, whether in the home, the hospital, the research institute, or the epidemiological office with its attendant computer, one of the three major problems is that of neoplastic disease. In the time of our grandparents and great grandparents the predominant cause of illness and of death was infective disease. Now, with our greater knowledge of the biology of infecting micro-organisms, and with the application of that knowledge in terms of hygiene, the control of public health, prevention both by hygienic measures and by immunization, and treatment especially by the use of the potent chemotherapeutic and antibiotic agents which have come into use during the past 30 years, we are able to hold infectious disease more or less at bay. In its place as causes of morbidity and of mortality in a population which is enjoying a greater measure of longevity, we are faced with the degenerative diseases, particularly those of the cardiovascular system, coronary infarction, and cerebrovascular accidents, and with neoplastic disease.

This book is directed to a discussion of the general features of this last group of diseases and is oriented towards the effects of neoplastic disease in the one species, *Homo sapiens*, with which we are all personally concerned as members, and which the medical profession is dedicated to serve by the use of its special skills, experience, and understanding.

Tumours are extremely common. If a careful search is made of the body of any individual, one or more small overgrowths of tissue will be found. Small excrescences on the skin, patches of pigmented cells in the epidermis, spherical nodules of cells in the suprarenal or kidney, fibrous nodules in the muscle of the uterus, all these may be found, and

INTRODUCTION

could, by the strictest criteria, be designated as benign new growths, tumours *sensu stricto*. At the other end of the scale are the rapidly progressive, expanding, infiltrating, and metastasizing tumours which are such obvious and tragic manifestations of uncontrolled cell overgrowth. Study of the Mortality Bills shows that about 1 in 5 of all deaths is due to malignant disease, and, allowing for the successful treatment of many cases, it can be estimated that between 1 in 3 and 1 in 4 individuals will develop some form of malignant disease during their lifetime.

The treatment and prevention of disease are still, and are likely to remain for some time, at least partly empirical, but the practice of Scientific Medicine, with its greater prospects for accurate diagnosis, treatment, and prognosis, depends on an understanding of the biological processes of neoplasia. At present we are on the surface of the corpus of knowledge of this subject, but we should use our accumulated learning as a basis on which to exercise the pragmatic arts of healing. In this small volume I shall consider the varieties of malignant disease, the effects of tumours, both locally and generally, histological and cytological features, the concepts of the precancerous state and of regression and progression, and a number of factors which are concerned with the development and growth of clinically apparent tumours.

CHAPTER II
DEFINITIONS AND CLASSIFICATION

DEFINITIONS

EVERYONE who is professionally concerned with neoplastic disease whether as a clinician concerned with the management of patients, as a pathologist dealing with the laboratory investigation of tumours, or as a research worker trying to advance the sum of human knowledge on this great problem, is aware in his own mind what he means by a tumour, but it is extraordinarily difficult to set out a definition which is acceptable to all users and which is applicable to all forms of neoplastic disease. Etymologically, the word 'tumour' and the suffix '-oma' both connote the presence of a mass of tissue. The alternative term 'neoplasm' literally means new growth. Both these terms are useful in their way, but there are many swellings both acute and chronic which have no connexion with the diseases which we understand under the term 'tumour'. Similarly, there may be new growth of bone or other tissues in situations in which they are not usually found in response to irritative stimuli, but these are reactive phenomena, metaplasias, and again not to be considered in the same group as the 'true tumours'.

It will perhaps be easier to consider some of the characters of lesions accepted as neoplastic disease and to accept that definitive concepts may be available for individual tumour types, but that at present a completely satisfactory overall set of criteria cannot be set forth. The first characteristic of tumours is that there is excessive growth of cells, an increased number of cells of one or more particular types is present at one or several situations. This growth of cells is excessive but is not necessarily unduly rapid. No tumour in the adult has been described which consistently increases in size as rapidly as does the foetus in utero, and the cell duplication essential to tissue growth often proceeds at a greater rate in tissues such as the intestinal mucosa than in the apparently most rapidly growing tumours. We must therefore qualify the character of excessive growth by the stipulation that the cell multiplication is out of control in the case of most malignant tumours, and only partially controlled in the case of benign tumours. In normal physiological circumstances the size of an organ and the number of cells which it contains remain approximately constant. This constancy is effected by control mechanisms which regulate the mitotic cycle of the cells of the tissue in such a way as to maintain the optimum number of cells. The exact nature of these mechanisms is uncertain. There is evidence that chemicals may be released by differentiated cells which hold in check future mitotic activity but allow cell growth to replace cells which are lost. There is also some evidence to support an alternative hypothesis that the control of cell numbers is part of the responsibility of the reticulo-endothelial system by a somewhat more complex mechanism. Further controls are exerted more generally by the overall endocrine control of the functions of the body. In neoplastic disease these controls are, to a greater or lesser extent, negated or deviated.

This modified concept of the nature of neoplastic disease must be further qualified by the caveat that a simple aetiological factor is not known. For example, in untreated pernicious anaemia there is an overgrowth consisting mainly of erythroid cells which are abnormal. The haematologist recognizes them as megaloblasts rather than as normoblasts. These cells may occupy a major part of the bone-marrow as do the atypical cells of leukaemia and may be found in the liver and spleen. We know, however, that pernicious anaemia is a deficiency disease due to a lack of absorption of vitamin B_{12} and the condition is not classified as a tumour. In the case of overactivity of the parathyroid, tumour-like masses of fibrous tissue may be found in the bones. These may resemble some forms of bone tumour histologically but are recognized as a manifestation of hormonal excess. It is possible that further disease entities which are presently regarded as neoplastic in nature will one day prove to be due to an excess of, or a deficiency of, some as yet unrecognized body components.

The next major characteristic is shown by tumours which are claimed as malignant and comprises the capacity to invade and to metastasize. Normally cells remain in the organ or part in which their function lies, as a consequence of local controls, and do not extend either locally or distantly. In the case of many malignant tumours extension and invasion of surrounding tissues are obvious and characteristic properties and the limit of extension may be difficult or impossible to detect. Distant extension, metastasis, is also usually eventually seen in malignant disease and will be discussed at length in CHAPTER IV. Local extension and metastasis are, however, not necessary criteria for the identification of malignant tumours. Many growths are recognized and treated before that stage is reached with results which are gratifying both to the surgeon and to the patient.

BENIGN AND MALIGNANT

The first and, from the point of view of the clinician and of the patient, the most important subdivision of tumours is into those which are benign and those which are malignant. This distinction is often made

DEFINITIONS AND CLASSIFICATION

on the basis of histological criteria, but it is an essentially clinical subdivision. A malignant tumour is one which will, if left untreated, spread locally and perhaps distantly, and will probably cause the death of the patient. A benign tumour, on the other hand, is one which proliferates locally and usually remains circumscribed. The growth of the tumour is usually slow, and the ill effects on the patient are related to the site, size, and physical presence of the lesion, and not to direct invasion of vital structures. A typical malignant tumour is carcinoma of the lung, which spreads, in the lung tissue, to the local lymph-nodes and metastasizes to the brain, bones, liver, adrenals, and other organs; in a distressingly high proportion of cases the patient dies as a direct consequence of the tumour. In contrast, a typical benign tumour is the uterine fibroid which forms a spherical mass in the myometrium: it can be shelled out from its capsule and may remain in situ for many years without causing any apparent ill effects.

These two definitions are excellent in their way, but, like so many definitions, do not tell the whole story. In many instances there is a clear-cut distinction between benign tumours and malignant tumours in the clinical course of the disease, in the anatomical appearance of the tumour, and in the histological appearances of the neoplastic tissue. In general the cells of benign tumours are well differentiated and can readily be identified and classified according to their origin from normal cells which they resemble closely. Malignant cells, on the other hand, are less well differentiated and show increased mitotic activity. The edge of a benign tumour is usually clear cut while that of a malignant tumour is less well defined, and careful examination will show finger-like projections of cells extending irregularly into the surrounding tissue. There is, however, a zone between benign and malignant. Some tumours have characters which belong to both groups and it may be difficult to define in a word the nature of the lesion.

Many examples of lesions of this type can be given. The common basal-cell carcinoma of the skin extends and invades locally but rarely metastasizes. Some sarcomata are prone to recur locally if incompletely removed but metastasize only after a prolonged period. Atypical hyperplasia of the endometrium is sometimes seen in women with an excess of circulating oestrogens, and the equivocal opinion, 'not carcinoma, but better out', may be given (*Fig.* 1). The group of disorders designated 'carcinoma-in-situ' or the precancerous states, which will be considered in CHAPTER VI, also fall into this group.

It must be accepted that there is a zone of transition in behaviour between the obviously benign and the unequivocally malignant. In this zone some lesions, such as basal-cell carcinoma, are well defined, and can be described by simple verbal formulae. Other lesions are less well defined and the work of the surgical histologist becomes much more 'clinical'. He is called upon to help his surgical colleagues to formulate a plan of treatment based on all the available information and on an appraisal of the likely consequences of the various possible modes of therapy. In such cases a more general opinion is necessary, but in my view such terms as 'benign metastasizing goitre' and 'locally malignant' should be eschewed and instead an explicit clinicopathological term or phrase should be used.

The boundary between benign and malignant or between 'grades' of malignancy is man-made, and is often a matter of semantic difference only. Some pathologists do not recognize the existence of benign tumours of fibrous tissue and consider all to be fibrosarcomata. This is acceptable as long as it is understood that some of the lesions in this group are curable by simple local excision. Similarly, there is a lesion of the bladder which is readily controlled by simple local surgical measures. In the U.K. this lesion is usually called 'papilloma', but in many centres of the U.S.A. it is called 'papillary carcinoma of the bladder, grade I'. The difference is purely one of words. The therapy used and the results achieved are identical, because in each case both the surgeon and the pathologist give the same connotation to the expression used.

CLASSIFICATION

An essential part of the understanding of any group of phenomena is the recognition that subgroups can be formed on the basis of several sets of criteria. The chemical elements are divisible into the groups of the Periodic Table in a manner which allows the chemist to predict the properties of an element from its position in the classification. At an even more fundamental level the particles of nuclear physics are subdivided into groups depending on their various properties. In the case of pathological entities an ideal classification will comprise criteria relating to site, aetiology, appearance, and behaviour, so that groups of lesions carrying similar clinical implications can be recognized in order to facilitate both treatment and prognosis. In the case of tumours, the factors concerned in aetiology are for the most part unknown, and for clinical purposes the aetiological component of the classification is of little value. Classification by site, tumours of stomach, lung, bone, brain, etc., is of great clinical interest, but is less important in a pathological context where the basis for most classifications is a combination of the tissue of origin and an estimate of the expected behaviour.

Two methods of classifying tumours will be mentioned. The first is a conventional pathological grouping with emphasis on the type of cell from which the tumour is thought to have arisen; the second is a clinicopathological subclassification of tumours of particular types and sites which is useful in assessing behaviour in the family of neoplasms and the prognosis in an individual and in comparing therapeutic procedures.

DEFINITIONS AND CLASSIFICATION

A PATHOLOGICAL CLASSIFICATION

The basis of this classification is firstly the distinction between benign and malignant tumours on the basis of the expected natural course of the disease, and secondly the nature of the cell of origin. One such classification is given in *Table I*. It corresponds generally to those given by other writers and is for the most part self-explanatory, but a few comments and explanations may be helpful.

A division into benign and malignant is given, but five lesions are placed on the line of division. Basal-cell carcinoma of the skin is by its nature intermediate between the benign and the malignant neoplasms (*Figs.* 2, 3, 4). Phaeochromocytoma, the catecholamine-secreting tumour of the adrenal and the organ of Zuckerkandl, and the carcinoid tumours which arise in the argentaffin tissues of the gastro-intestinal tract are also intermediate in behaviour and both may on occasion metastasize. In the case of osteoclastoma, the giant-cell tumour of bone, both benign and malignant variants may exist without a clear histological demarcation between them. Finally, chorio-adenoma destruens is recognized by some pathologists as being intermediate in behaviour between hydatidiform mole and chorionepithelioma. In some cases, especially tumours of the connective tissues, a line has been added connecting the benign and malignant forms of tumour. This indicates that there is a range of histological and clinical types with gradations of behaviour.

Two benign lesions are noted as tumours of striated muscle. The first of these, the rhabdomyoma, is extremely rare and its existence is doubted; the second, granular-cell myoblastoma, is seen in the tongue and upper respiratory tract. The cells do not resemble muscle cells closely but have histological and cytological features which suggest that they take origin from striated muscle cells.

The hamartomata lie in the borderland between congenital malformations and tumours. Many of the small cutaneous lesions which consist of small capillary and venous blood spaces are present as a result of maldevelopment of part of the vascular system, and exist firstly as potential tumours in the form of closed blood spaces which become clinically apparent when they dilate and fill with blood. Other lesions in this group consist of conglomerations of tissue elements which are potentially part of the organs in which they arise but are arranged in a disorderly manner as in the bronchial hamartoma which comprises glandular elements embedded in a dense mass of cartilage. Most commonly the hamartoma is a benign lesion, but occasionally malignant transformation may occur.

The embryonic tumours occur mostly in children and consist of elements thought to represent embryonic anlagen of the tissues and organs in which they arise. They are usually malignant and often include bizarre cells showing modes of differentiation such as striated muscle which are not seen in the adult tissue or organ.

Table I.—A Pathological Classification of Tumours

Cell of Origin	Benign	Malignant
Epithelial		
Squamous	Papilloma	Carcinoma
Glandular	Adenoma	Adenocarcinoma
Transitional	Papilloma ←————→ Carcinoma	
Basal	Basal-cell carcinoma	
Pigmented cells	Benign melanoma (naevus)	Malignant melanoma
Glial cells		
Astrocytes		Astrocytoma
Ependyma		Ependymoma
Oligodendroglia		Oligodendroglioma
Primitive glial cells		Ependymoblastoma
		Medulloblastoma
Nerve cells	Ganglioneuroma	Neuroblastoma
	Phaeochromocytoma	
Connective-tissue cells		
Fibrous tissue	Fibroma ←————→ Fibrosarcoma	
Myxoid tissue	Myxoma ←————→ Myxosarcoma	
Smooth muscle	Leiomyoma ←————→ Leiomyosarcoma	
Striated muscle	Rhabdomyoma	Rhabdomyosarcoma
	Granular-cell myoblastoma	
Cartilage	Chondroma	Chondrosarcoma
	Benign chondroblastoma	
Bone	Osteoma	Osteogenic sarcoma
	Osteoid osteoma	
	←————Osteoclastoma————→	
Fat	Lipoma	Liposarcoma
Synovium	Synovioma ←————→ Synovial sarcoma	
Vessels	Haemangioma	Angiosarcoma
	Lymphangioma	
	Glomangioma	
	Haemangiopericytoma	
Nerve sheath	Neurofibroma	Neurofibrosarcoma
Notochord	Chondroma	Malignant chondroma
Haemopoietic tissues		
Lymphoid cells	Follicular lymphoma	Lymphosarcoma
		Reticulosarcoma
		Hodgkin's disease
		Lymphatic leukaemia
Myeloid cells		Myeloid leukaemia
		Monocytic leukaemia
Plasma cells		Myelomatosis
Erythroid cells		Primary polycythaemia
Special classes of tumours		
Hamartomata		
Embryonic tumours		Nephroblastoma
		Hepatoblastoma
		Botryoid sarcoma
Argentaffin tissue	Carcinoid	
Mixed tumours		Carcinosarcoma
		Mixed salivary tumour
		Mixed mesodermal tumour
Chemoreceptor	Chemodectoma	Alveolar soft-part sarcoma
Foetal tissue	Hydatidiform mole	Chorionepithelioma
	Chorio-adenoma destruens	
Germ cells	Teratoma	Teratocarcinoma
		Seminoma
		Disgerminoma

DEFINITIONS AND CLASSIFICATION

Mixed tumours are characterized by the presence of cells showing differentiation in two or more ways. It is common for connective-tissue neoplasms to show more than one type of connective-tissue cell, but these are usually designated as osteochondroma, fibrolipoma, chondrofibromyxoma, or under some such combined descriptive title, and it is accepted that there is a marked capacity for such dual differentiation in cells of this type. More complex structural mixtures are seen in the mixed salivary tumour (*Fig.* 5) and in the mixed mesodermal tumour of the endometrium and in carcinosarcoma (*Fig.* 6). In the case of the common mixed salivary tumour the lesion comprises epithelial and myoepithelial elements set in a matrix of mucoid and chondroid tissue. It is probable that the lesion is wholly epithelial in nature and that the apparent connective-tissue element is derived from specialized myoepithelial cells which lie at the periphery of salivary gland ducts and acini. The mixed mesodermal tumour of the endometrium may contain diverse mesenchymal elements such as bone, cartilage, fat, and striated muscle, and there may also be areas of patent adenocarcinoma. The explanation of this lesion lies in the developmental history of the uterus which derives its origin from the fused lower ends of the Müllerian ducts which are mesodermal structures. The lining of the uterus, despite its epithelial character, consists of mesodermal cells, and, in the case of neoplastic change, these can assume modes of differentiation typical of both connective-tissue and of epithelial cells. This tumour is, therefore, a true carcinosarcoma consisting of neoplastic cells of both epithelial and connective-tissue type of monoblastic origin. Most other so-called 'carcinosarcomata' are misnamed because of an unusual spindle-cell type of carcinoma cell in one part of a tumour or because of metaplastic change in the connective-tissue stroma of a carcinoma.

The three grades of tumour of foetal tissue—hydatidiform mole, chorio-adenoma destruens, and chorionepithelioma—are unique in that, while they are seen clinically in a female, they are tumours of the trophoblastic tissue of another individual, her foetus. The chorionepithelioma of the testis, the only form of this tumour found in the male, is a special derivative of testicular teratoma. The wide range of differentiation in this tumour can include trophoblastic elements (*see Fig.* 16) (*see also* CHAPTER XV). Consideration of the detailed pathology of these tumours involves not only the usual neoplastic characters but also the complications added by the different genetic nature of the host and tumour cells. It is possible that this difference and the mechanism of transplant rejection are involved in the unusually good response of these lesions to chemotherapeutic measures.

The teratomata, benign and malignant, are also unique in tumour pathology. The most exacting definition of the teratoma is that it is a tumour comprising tissue elements of all three germ layers, ectoderm, mesoderm, and endoderm, although in an individual lesion it may not be possible to make a positive identification of all three types of tissue, for example in struma ovarii where all the tumour tissue appears to be of thyroid type. These tumours are seen mainly in the gonads and less often in other situations. Many are benign, but those that are malignant may show their malignant propensity either directly as a teratocarcinoma or by the development of a malignant potential in one element of the tumour, e.g., carcinoma arising in the skin in a dermoid cyst of the ovary. The general pathology of teratomata shows features which differ from those of other tumours and I have added a separate chapter, the only chapter on a single tumour type, to this volume (CHAPTER XV).

A PROGNOSTIC CLASSIFICATION

When patients with neoplastic disease come to operation, four anatomical parameters are available for the assessment of the future course of the disease. These are: the histological nature of the tumour, the anatomical extent of the tumour, the presence of lymph-node metastases, and the presence of distant metastases. The role of the histological grading of tumours will be discussed in CHAPTER V and is obviously relevant to the other gradings used.

Several years ago Dukes suggested that the prognosis in cancer of the colon and rectum could be assessed by identification of four categories of increasingly poor prognosis. His group A comprises tumours involving the gut wall only, group B those which have invaded through the gut wall, group C, sometimes subdivided into CI and CII and CIII, those which have involved local and distant lymph-nodes, and group D those in which there are distant metastases. This method of subdivision is now being superseded by the internationally accepted TNM system, in which three components are used: T referring to the size and local extension of the primary tumour; N referring to the presence and extent of lymph-node metastases, and M referring to the presence or absence of distant metastases. The criteria for assessment under each component vary according to the site and type of lesion, for example, component T in the case of breast carcinoma includes information on the degree of fixation to deep structures and to skin, while in the case of gastric carcinoma, extension through and along the muscle of the stomach wall and invasion of adjacent viscera are important.

This type of classification is designed for a specific end, in this case, assessment of the prognosis, and can be very useful both in assessing an individual patient and also in ensuring that two series of cases consist of comparable lesions.

CHAPTER III

CLINICOPATHOLOGICAL CORRELATION IN TUMOURS

TUMOURS produce symptoms and signs which are detectable by clinical interrogation and examination and as the result of special laboratory, radiological, and other examinations. They also, in time, may cause the death of the host patient. The symptoms and signs and the eventual fatal outcome are not simply a function of the size of a tumour. The average weight of an adult male is some 70 kg. (140 lb.), and a tumour which weighs more than a small fraction of this, 2 kg. (4 lb.) or 3 per cent of the body-weight, is regarded as very large. In most cases the mass of tumour is only a few grammes yet it causes symptoms and can be lethal. It is a legitimate part of our concern with the general pathology of tumours to discuss the available information concerning the ways in which the effects of tumours are produced. A division into local and general effects will be made and a discussion of the several types of interaction will be given. It must be remembered, however, that in any patient the clinical manifestations will be the result of all the effects of the primary tumour, and of the secondary growths emanating from it, both local and general. The local effects may be due to a primary tumour arising in the part affected or may be due to a secondary deposit from a lesion which is producing apparent or inapparent local effects elsewhere in the body.

LOCAL EFFECTS

Before the introduction of antibiotics and chemotherapeutic agents, it was an aphorism of general medicine that any symptom with which a patient presented and any sign which could be elicited could be due to syphilis. Today it is equally true to state that any symptoms and signs can be due to tumour. Any part of the body may be affected by neoplastic disease; the local effect will depend on the site and on the way in which the tumour interferes with normal form and function.

TUMOUR MASS

A tumour may become apparent simply as an abnormal swelling in the tissues. This is most often the case when the lesion is in a superficial situation: tumours of the skin and of the breast, swelling of the testis, nodules in subcutaneous bones such as the skull or the tibia may be noticed simply because they are swellings in abnormal situations. Less often tissues of deep structures may cause no symptoms but be detected on casual or routine palpation; a uterine fibroid may be noted when the abdomen is felt although it has otherwise caused no symptoms. Occasionally a large tumour may come to notice because of a non-specific feeling of an abnormal internal mass, perhaps because it is pulling on ligaments which are normally lax. Superficial tumours, especially of the skin, may be subject to minor trauma and become infected and ulcerated.

IRRITATION

The presence of tumour tissue may have an irritative effect on adjacent structures. The nature of this effect depends on the normal function of the part irritated as the effect of over-stimulation is to produce over-action. Nerves may be irritated by the direct action of infiltrating tumour tissue or by stimulation when they are stretched or compressed by tumour in a confined space, or by the fibrous stroma which commonly forms around tumour cells. This over-stimulation of nerve-fibres results in an excessive series of impulses passing centrally. These are interpreted as pain which is referred to the areas of normal distribution of the nerves concerned. This is a common and important mechanism by which pain is produced in cancer, but it is not the only one. Pain may also be the result of obstruction of hollow viscera with distension proximal to the lesion.

The dry, brassy cough of lung cancer is due to an irritant effect on the nerve-endings which provide the afferent part of the cough reflex, and over-activity of the colonic musculature with consequent diarrhoea may similarly be due to irritation of nerve-endings. Secondary deposits of tumour frequently invade the bone-marrow and there their presence affects the haemopoietic mechanism, leading to a leuco-erythroblastic anaemia in which immature red and white cells are released into the circulation. The serous membranes, pleura, pericardium, and peritoneum, secrete a thin layer of lubricating fluid; if tumour deposits are present an excess of fluid is produced which is clinically detectable as effusion.

Direct stimulation of nerve-cells within the central nervous system leads to over-activity which is manifest as one or other of the various forms of epilepsy and is also detectable by changes in the pattern of the electro-encephalographic waves.

BLOOD-VESSELS

One of the commonest symptoms of neoplastic disease is haemorrhage which usually comes directly from the network of small blood-vessels which have developed in the stroma of the tumour. In most cases the tumour cells are relatively fragile and may break away leaving the thin-walled capillaries accessible to minor trauma. More serious haemorrhage, which may be grossly debilitating and even directly fatal, follows the invasion of the walls of vessels by tumour cells with resultant weakening and rupture. This haemorrhage may occur into any of the body cavities or into the substance of solid organs such as the brain.

Secondly, blood-vessels may be obstructed by pressure from tumour outside, and local intravascular coagulation, or, more rarely, by tumour growth within them. Obstruction leads to venous congestion with oedema which is an important cause of symptoms in brain tumours, and may also lead to gross swelling of the tissues of one or other limb, especially when it is combined with obstruction to the lymphatic vessels. Acute vascular obstruction due to torsion of a pedicle is seen in pedunculated tumours, particularly those which protrude into the abdominal cavity.

Finally, tumour tissue may grow inside a vessel and small fragments break off and become emboli. Most tumour emboli are small and the observable effect is the formation of metastatic deposits. Less commonly a large mass of tumour is released to produce the effect of a clinically apparent embolus which may be directly fatal. A rare expression of the uncommon myxoma of the auricle is obstruction of the mitral or tricuspid valves.

HOLLOW VISCERA

Most of the important organs of the body are hollow or depend for their function on the integrity of hollow ducts. These may be obstructed by the presence of tumour in three situations, outside the wall, in the wall, or in the lumen. Obstruction of a duct or viscus by pressure from without is most often seen in the case of small structures. The ureter may be obstructed by tumour in the retroperitoneal tissues of the pelvis; the bile-duct and pancreatic duct may be obstructed by tumour in the head of the pancreas or by lymph-nodes filled with metastases in the porta hepatis. The urethra may be obstructed by the mass of a carcinoma of the prostate surrounding it. Within the skull the flow of cerebrospinal fluid passes through narrow passages, the aqueduct of Sylvius and the foramina from the fourth ventricle, and an increase in size of the brain substance because of tumour or because of the associated oedema may obstruct these pathways giving rise to hydrocephalus.

Tumour in the wall of a viscus or duct is an important cause of obstruction; a colonic cancer can develop with its accompanying fibrosis as a ring stricture of the intestine producing complete or incomplete obstruction. Less often tumour deposits may affect the plexuses of nerves in the gut wall and, by depressing their function, produce a form of ileus, paralytic non-function of a section of gut which leads to an effective obstruction.

Obstruction of a hollow structure by the effect of tumour within the lumen is less common as the walls of such structures are usually sufficiently elastic to allow some flow of the contents. Bronchi are relatively stiff-walled structures and are often obstructed by carcinomata and by polypoid benign tumours. The ureter may be obstructed by a polypoid lesion of the renal pelvis and the bile-ducts may be obstructed by intraluminar tumour or by tumour tissue passing down the duct from a hepatic tumour. Obstruction of the intestine as the result of the presence of an intraluminal tumour is more often in the form of intussusception; a small polypoid lesion, often of lymphoid origin, forms the apex of the patch of infolded bowel.

In some cases distortion of the anatomy of the lumen of a hollow viscus is important. Uterine fibroids may reach considerable size and elongate and distort the uterine cavity with two effects: an increase in the area of endometrium and consequently an increase in the flow of menstrual blood; and the pathway for spermatozoa is altered with a consequent risk of infertility and of ectopic pregnancy. A similar distortion of the oesophagus may be seen in tumours of the mediastinum whether primary or secondary. The oesophagus is mobile and is pushed to one side by the enlarging tumour mass with resultant dysphagia.

Finally, necrosis of part of a tumour in a hollow viscus or destruction of the wall of the viscus may occur with perforation and release of the contents, usually intestinal or gastric, into the peritoneal cavity or into another space such as the bladder cavity or the vagina with secondary infection and sometimes the formation of a permanent fistula.

Rarely, the presence of a neoplasm in the wall of the intestine may interfere with the general function of the gut; malabsorption has, on occasion, been ascribed to the effect of an intestinal tumour arising in reticulo-endothelial cells.

INFECTION

Any tumour which is exposed to micro-organisms is liable to be infected, and, because of the lack of immune defences within the tumour, the neoplasm can undergo infective necrosis and ulceration. The obstructive effects of tumours also lead to stasis of fluid behind the obstruction providing a focus in which infection can readily occur. In the case of lung cancer there is an increase in frequency of onset during the periods when respiratory infection is common, the symptoms of the lesion become apparent when invasion of the lung behind the tumour with bacteria sets up a focus of pneumonia. There is also an increased liability to infection in general in patients with tumours partly due to bone-marrow replacement and depression and partly to depression and ultimate failure of the immune system.

DAMAGE TO VITAL STRUCTURES

As primary and secondary tumours grow the cells infiltrate between the normal cells of the part and cause extensive destruction of such cells. This may lead to a variety of clinical effects. Replacement of bone by neoplastic tissue weakens the structure and allows pathological fractures—breaks in the bone in response to minimal trauma—to occur. Destruction of nervous tissue leads to permanent loss of function, paralyses can be due to loss of nerve-cells in the motor pathways or to destruction of nerve-fibres, loss of sensory function may be due to loss of areas of sensory cortex or of parts of the sensory pathways, and psychological changes follow destruction of all or part of the frontal cortex.

Tumour in the bone-marrow, especially tumour of bone-marrow elements, leukaemia, and myelomatosis, can cause anaemia by replacing most of the available erythropoietic tissue. This anaemia is accompanied by a lack of blood platelets with the consequent risk of haemorrhage and by a lack of white blood cells which leads to an increased risk of infection.

GENERAL EFFECTS

The effect of a tumour on a patient, the clinical disease process which is produced, is often due to the local actions of tumour cells, but may also be due to the general effects of the tumour on metabolic processes.

PARASITIZATION

For many purposes a tumour may be regarded as a separate population of cells independent of, but parasitic upon, the host, and competing with him for nutrient and energy sources. As has been noted earlier, the mass of tumour tissue is usually small relative to the mass of the host, but occasionally, where a tumour has been allowed to grow to a very large size, the distribution of resources between the tumour and the host is detrimental to the latter. Occasional cases have been reported in which an ovarian cystadenocarcinoma, a uterine fibroid, or a lipoma has reached such a size that the host has suffered starvation in competition with the tumour.

TOXIC EFFECTS

As tumour cells metabolize they release into the circulation of the host waste products many of which are identical to those released by the host cells and which can be excreted, but some of which are the result of aberrant metabolic pathways in the tumour. To this load must be added the chemical products of breakdown of tumour cells, since examination of many tumours shows large numbers of necrotic cells. The combined effect of this increased load of toxic substances on the host is to depress his normal metabolic processes and to produce an overall state of inanition, which may be accentuated by faulty digestive and absorptive function and by the effects of concomitant infection.

HORMONES

The interactions of the various compounds secreted by the endocrine organs are of great importance in the study of tumours and will be discussed in a separate section (CHAPTER XII). It is sufficient here to comment that tumours arising in the several endocrine organs can secrete hormones which have a general effect on the metabolism of the body. Hyperactivity of the pituitary, thyroid, parathyroid, adrenal, both medulla and cortex, the ovary and testis, and the islet cells of the pancreas has been described as a consequence of neoplasia. A similar unusual endocrine phenomenon is the occurrence of polycythaemia in renal carcinomata and in some ovarian and adrenal tumours. In these cases it appears that the tumour cells produce erythropoietin which has the effect of stimulating normoblastic activity in the bone-marrow. It is not known whether the high haemoglobin levels associated with some vascular tumours of the central nervous system are due to a similar mechanism. The action of the smallest of these organs, the pituitary, may be reduced as a consequence of tumour compressing and destroying the gland substance. Endocrine activity is also seen in tumours of the widely distributed argentaffin cells. In most instances these are small lesions whose venous drainage is by the portal system and any hormones are detoxified in the liver, but in the presence of hepatic metastases the clinical effects of an excess of hydroxytryptamine become evident. Similar tumours are also seen in the bronchial mucosa where they form one class of bronchial adenomata. Placental gonadotrophins are produced both by chorionic tumours of the placenta and by the differentiated chorionic tissue which is to be found in teratomata, particularly of the testis. The association of myasthenia gravis with primary tumours of the thymus is probably due to a hormonal substance although this has not yet been identified and the association substantiated.

A non-specific hormone effect is seen in large connective-tissue tumours which are associated with hypoglycaemia. In some cases it has been suggested that the avidity of the tumour cells for glucose is sufficient to reduce the level of blood-sugar but there is also evidence that these tumours produce insulin-like substances.

Aberrant hormone production by tumours arising in cells not usually considered endocrine in nature has been described on a number of occasions. Most of these lesions have been lung tumours and the hormones have had the effect of the protein hormones of the pituitary and placenta. It is probable that this is some form of unblocking of genes specific for hormone production as immunofluorescent tests have failed to show evidence of placental antigens in tumours which are known to be elaborating placental hormones.

CLINICOPATHOLOGICAL CORRELATION IN TUMOURS

THROMBOPHLEBITIS MIGRANS

This curious and rare condition presents as repeated venous thromboses in varying parts of the body over a period. In some cases there is a diffuse disease of the vein walls analogous to Buerger's disease, thrombo-angiitis obliterans of the arteries. In other cases, and especially in younger individuals, the causative factor is a deep-seated tumour which often does not present any other clinical features. The mechanism underlying this phenomenon is uncertain.

IMMUNOSUPPRESSION

Patients suffering from tumours are more prone than normal individuals to develop intercurrent infection. In some part this is due to a general depression of bodily activities, but there is some evidence of a specific depression of the immune system. In lesions which involve the reticulo-endothelial system generally this suppression of immunity is well marked, and a variety of infections due to organisms normally of low pathogenicity, for example, torula and toxoplasma, may be seen. In the case of other tumours, it is arguable whether the deficiency in immunity which is seen is due to the presence of the tumour or is a causal factor in the production of the tumour.

SKIN DISEASES

The most obvious and, in some cases, the first clinical manifestation of neoplastic disease is seen in the skin. Skin lesions may form part of the syndrome in certain types of genetically determined neoplasms: the café-au-lait spots of the Peutz-Jegher syndrome of small intestinal polyposis and neurofibromatosis, and the sebaceous adenomata of tuberose sclerosis are examples of this association. A number of other non-specific dermal eruptions may be seen in patients with tumours, but there are also two conditions in which the presence of the eruptions should raise the suspicion of deep-seated tumour.

Dermatomyositis is a complex comprising a rash on the exposed parts of the body, muscle weakness, and fever. Most often this syndrome is due to abnormalities of the immune system, but occasionally, in up to about 10 per cent of cases, there is a neoplasm which acts as the precipitating factor. It is possible that in such cases the systemic lesions are an allergic response to the presence of tumour antigens and the tumour may be very small.

The skin lesion acanthosis nigricans is associated with carcinoma of the gastro-intestinal tract in almost 90 per cent of cases seen in adults. The dermatological manifestation is of hypertrophy and pigmentation of the skin, especially in the neck, axilla, and groin, and also involving the umbilicus and nipples. Later warty papillomata arise in the affected areas, but these are local skin lesions, and not secondary deposits. The tumours which are associated with acanthosis nigricans are usually highly malignant and spread rapidly.

CARCINOMATOUS NEUROPATHY

Neurological symptoms and signs in patients suffering from malignant disease are most often due to the presence of metastases in the brain, spinal cord, or nerves. Occasionally, however, cases are described in which there is evidence of degenerative disease of the central nervous system and of peripheral nerves. The principal clinical forms which these conditions take are: cerebellar disorders, ataxia, and vertigo; sensory neuropathy with sensory loss, motor neuropathy with wasting and weakness of muscles, a combined motor and sensory neuropathy; epileptiform attacks or psychological changes. In other cases there is a defect in neuromuscular transmission in voluntary muscles, and in others again a progressive multifocal demyelination in the cerebrum.

Histological studies have shown that these disorders are not due to the presence of malignant cells, although in some cases a pleocytosis in the cerebrospinal fluid suggests that there must be some local factor. The mechanism is unknown although it is possible that an allergic reaction similar to that postulated for dermatomyositis may be involved. This complication of tumours is rare, less than 1 per cent of all patients with tumours show these clinical phenomena. The direct relationship of the neurological disorders to the presence of the primary tumour is shown by the regression of symptoms in some cases when the primary tumour is removed.

CHAPTER IV
THE SPREAD OF TUMOURS

A PRIMARY characteristic of tumours is that their growth is uncontrolled or partially controlled, and that if untreated they tend to increase in size and to spread. In the case of benign tumours the increase in size is relatively slow and space is made for the tumour by pushing the surrounding tissues aside and distorting them. This extension tends to evoke a reaction in the surrounding tissues; a fibrous capsule is often formed around a benign tumour, and at operation it may be possible to incise the capsule and to enucleate the tumour. The extension of benign tumours may produce surgical problems if the lesion lies close to vital structures, but as a pathological manifestation of the neoplastic disease it is relatively trivial. In malignant tumours, on the other hand, the spread of the lesion is of the most vital importance, as it determines the clinical manifestations of the disease, the prognosis, and the therapeutic measures which may be possible. The remainder of this chapter will deal with the problem of the spread of malignant tumours.

LOCAL SPREAD

In contrast to the typical benign tumour, the malignant neoplasm does not increase in size simply by pushing aside the adjacent normal tissues. The cells of a malignant tumour are less constrained in their growth than those of a benign lesion and can infiltrate between the surrounding tissue cells, separating groups of cells and forming finger-like projections which may extend widely into the surrounding tissues. These extensions are well seen in breast carcinoma and the puckering of the skin as if by the claws of a crab has given the common name 'cancer' to malignant tumours. Extension beyond the apparent limits of the tumour may be widespread, an observation well recognized by surgeons who are accustomed to make extensive excisions of malignant tissue with a surrounding layer of normal tissue. This local extension may involve many structures and can be responsible for many of the clinical manifestations of cancers. In rare cases a tumour may extend in continuity over several parts of the body and so produce its entire clinical picture. More usually, however, there is distant spread of the tumour without continuity. This phenomenon we call 'metastasis'.

METASTASIS

Metastasis, the implantation of viable growing cells in parts of the body distant from the primary tumour, is characteristic of malignant neoplasms and is most often the factor which determines the eventual death of the patient. Metastases can occur anywhere in the body, although there are some sites where metastatic tumour is more common, and can arise by a variety of mechanisms. For a metastasis to occur a number of conditions must be satisfied. Cells must be able to break away from the primary tumour; a mechanism of transportation must be available for them to be carried to the secondary site; once in the secondary site they must be arrested; and finally they must be capable of growing in the secondary site because of the intrinsic growth capacity of the tumour cells, and because of the suitability of the site at which they lodge.

SITES OF METASTASIS

The most common sites at which metastases are found are the lung, liver, bones, brain, lymph-nodes, and skin. Secondary deposits in small organs such as the adrenals, gonads, thyroid, and pituitary are possibly less common because of the statistically small chance of a few circulating tumour cells being arrested in such situations. In the case of some larger structures, such as the skeletal muscle, secondary deposits are rare; the reason for this is unknown but may be related to the speed of blood-flow through these structures or to the high metabolic activity, with concomitant high oxygen tension, and possibly the accumulation of lactic acid. The major organs of metastasis, the lung and liver, have a blood-supply from the right side of the heart and the portal vein respectively, which carries little oxygen, which may favour metastasis, and in the bone-marrow there are pools of relatively stagnant blood which could also be depleted of oxygen. The differential distributions of secondary deposits is one of the very many problems in tumour pathology which remain to be solved.

MECHANISMS OF METASTASIS

Tumour cells can be carried along any tubular structure in the body which is big enough to accommodate the cell and which contains fluid. The most common routes by which metastases are spread are the bloodstream and the lymphatic system, but extension can also take place across the pleural and peritoneal cavities, through the meningeal spaces, along the ureter, through the uterine cavity and the Fallopian tubes, down the bile-ducts, and across the vagina. Metastasis by way of the gastro-intestinal tract is uncommon, possibly because of the digestive enzymes which may be expected to be inimical to the safe passage of malignant cells.

BLOOD-BORNE METASTASIS

Many malignant tumours have the property of invading the walls of small blood-vessels and groups of tumour cells can be seen lying within the lumen of a vessel bathed by the circulating blood. This is particularly apparent in sarcomata and in the case of hypernephroma of the kidney which often grows as a tongue of tissue extending into the renal vein and the inferior vena cava. Small groups of tumour cells can break away and be carried in the blood-stream to distant parts of the body. Cytological examination of blood samples has shown that circulating tumour cells are very frequently present in patients with malignant tumours, but that the presence of such cells does not inevitably presage metastasis. The small groups of tumour cells are carried in the blood-stream until they are blocked in a capillary which is too small for them to traverse, or until they become attached to the wall of a blood-vessel in a situation of slow blood-flow.

The distribution of blood-borne metastases generally follows the pattern of blood-flow. Primary lung tumours release cells into the pulmonary veins, the cells are carried through the left side of the heart to the systemic arteries, and metastatic deposits are seen in the brain, bones, liver, kidney, and adrenals. Tumours of systemic organs whose venous drainage is to the superior or inferior venae cavae release cells which are carried to the lungs, where they settle in the pulmonary capillaries and produce pulmonary secondary deposits, which become rounded or are destroyed. The abdominal organs of the gastro-intestinal tract have a special venous drainage to the liver by the portal system and tend to produce blood-borne metastases in that organ. The tendency for tumours of the right side of the colon to metastasize to the right side of the liver and for tumours of the left side of the colon to metastasize to the left side of the liver has been attributed to the tendency for the relatively large tumour cells to remain on one or other side of the stream of blood in the portal vein and then to enter the corresponding intrahepatic branch of the vein.

In some cases, however, the pattern of blood-flow is not followed, and blood-borne metastases may arise which are carried by apparently different routes. Cerebral secondary deposits may be seen from tumours whose blood supply is systemic in the absence of lung lesions. Very rarely these are due to paradoxical embolism through a patent right to left communication in the heart. More often they are the result of cells which are capable of passing through the pulmonary capillary bed without lodging there, or are the result of cells released from small, undetectable, clumps of tumour cells growing in the lung substance. A further anomalous form of blood-borne metastasis involves the plexuses of veins which lie around the vertebral column and in the pelvis. The blood-flow in these veins is not in a constant direction and metastasis can occur within the system. It is possible that metastases from the thyroid directly to the vertebral bodies may be along these channels.

LYMPHATIC METASTASES

All organs and tissues except the central nervous system are served by elements of the lymphatic system. Material is collected and carried by small lymph channels to the lymph-nodes, collections of lymphoid tissue situated in various sites throughout the body. The cells of epithelial tumours are particularly prone to invade the lymph-vessels and to spread first to the local lymph-nodes, where they are characteristically first seen in the peripheral sinuses, and later, centripetally, to other groups elsewhere in the body. The drainage of lymph follows a pattern as does the venous drainage and the location of initial lymph-node metastases is determined by this drainage, which in turn indicates the likely sites of metastasis to which the surgeon should direct his attention. In most cases the neoplastic cells are carried as emboli through the lymphatics although occasionally permeation in continuity may be seen.

Eventually the lymph is passed from the system of lymph-nodes to the venous system by way of the thoracic duct, and blood-borne metastasis may be added to lymphatic metastasis if the cells reach this part of the lymphatic system. Apparently paradoxical lymphatic spread may occur if lymph-vessels are blocked by tumour or by inflammation, and tumour cells may be carried centrifugally to distal nodes rather than to those which are more proximal.

COELOMIC SURFACES

Four of the body cavities, the two pleural cavities, the peritoneum, and the pericardial cavity, form potential spaces lined by a mesothelial layer of cells. If tumours of the organs which lie in these cavities reach and extend through the covering mesothelium, cells may be released into the space and can then settle elsewhere to produce secondary deposits. This mode of spread is most common in the peritoneal cavity where deposits of gastro-intestinal tumours are frequently seen in the pelvic peritoneum and on the pelvic organs, especially the ovaries. Occasionally there is widespread dissemination of tumour throughout the cavity and tumour cells may develop which can survive suspended freely in peritoneal fluid. This phenomenon is seen more often in animal material and the 'ascites form' of many experimental tumours is a useful controllable model.

In human material the peritoneal cavity is more often the route of spread of neoplastic cells and secondary tumour masses in the pelvis may present clinically without there being overt signs of the primary lesion in the upper abdomen. Transpleural spread from primary lung cancer is a relatively late phenomenon in the course of the disease but is seen more often following the development of primary tumours of the pleura or secondary tumours in the lung. A possible explanation of this is that primary tumours tend to spread centripetally by the lymphatics and veins towards the mediastinum, while secondary tumours, which reach the lung by the arterial tree, are passing centrifugally towards the pleura.

SPREAD ALONG THE URETER AND BLADDER

Tumours of the kidney, either of the renal pelvis or of the renal substance, may spread down the ureter to form secondary deposits in the bladder. This spread may be by way of the lumen of the ureter, or possibly along lymphatic channels in the wall of the ureter. In the latter case lesions in the bladder wall may be expected. Primary bladder tumours release cells into the urine, but these are probably not viable, and secondary tumours in the bladder wall are more likely to arise by direct implantation as the walls of an empty bladder come together.

SPREAD THROUGH THE FEMALE GENITAL TRACT

There is a continuously patent passage between the fimbriated end of the Fallopian tube and the exterior by way of the uterus and vagina. Cells from carcinomata of the uterus and ovary may pass along the Fallopian tube to produce secondary deposits in the ovary and uterus respectively. Carcinoma of the cervix at the lower end of the uterus commonly extends into the vagina, usually by direct extension, but sometimes by the lymphatics of the vaginal wall or across the vaginal cavity.

SPREAD BY THE BILE-DUCTS

Tumours within the liver may invade the intrahepatic bile-ducts and spread by way of the bile-duct system to the common bile-duct and gall-bladder. This is a most unusual mode of spread which I have seen on only one occasion.

SPREAD IN THE CEREBROSPINAL FLUID

It is a characteristic of primary tumours of the central nervous system that they do not, except in very unusual circumstances, spread outside the confines of the skull and spinal cord. Cells may, however, be released from gliomata into the cerebrospinal fluid and be carried to other sites, most often the surface of the spinal cord.

A similar mode of spread is seen in connective-tissue tumours of the meninges and nerve-sheaths within the skull and spinal canal, and after deposition of tumour cells from other parts of the body. In these cases, and also in tumours of the reticulo-endothelial system, a thin layer of tumour cells may lie in the pia arachnoid, producing a 'malignant meningitis'.

OTHER CONSIDERATIONS

Discussion of the problem of the spread of tumours would be incomplete without mention of some relevant associated topics.

RETICULO-ENDOTHELIAL TUMOURS

These lesions arise in the lymphoid, myeloid, and reticular tissues, and may spread by continuity or as lymphatic or blood-borne metastases. The appearance of circulating tumour cells of this system, the haematological entity of leukaemia, has been interpreted as a tumour with circulating metastases. I think, however, that a better concept is that in the leukaemias the malignant cells have developed the ability to survive while floating freely in the circulating blood and that this should be regarded as a separate phenomenon distinct from metastasis.

DORMANT CANCER CELLS

Most often the course of malignant disease is a steady inexorable progress from initiation to the death of the patient, unless it can be arrested by therapeutic measures. Sometimes a tumour is recognized and treated and the patient remains well for many years until a crop of secondary deposits develops. In such cases there is a modification of the usual mode of metastasis. Malignant cells are spread in the body by the blood-stream or the lymphatics, they settle among the normal tissues and remain viable, but do not multiply. This stage of dormancy may be determined by the nature of the tumour cell or by the action of controlling factors, which are probably immunological in nature, in the host tissue. At some later time, for reasons not yet known, the multiplicative capacity of the cells increases, and local control is lost with the result that clinically evident late metastases occur.

UNDETECTABLE PRIMARY TUMOURS

It is not uncommon for a patient to present clinically with evidence of a space-occupying lesion which is found on histological examination to be metastatic. Subsequent clinical and radiological examination of the patient may fail to reveal the site of the primary lesion, which may only be detected after an exhaustive autopsy, or may not even be found then. There are two ways in which this situation can arise. The primary tumour may be intrinsically slowly growing locally, yet have a well-developed capacity for metastasis, or the growth of the primary lesion may be held in check by local immunological activity, which may indeed result in the obliteration of the primary lesion, while the secondary deposits in an area less well endowed with immunological capacity may be able to grow. In such cases surgical excision of the secondary deposit may give great benefit to the patient and may even effect a clinical cure.

CHAPTER V
DIFFERENTIATION, DEDIFFERENTIATION, AND TUMOUR HISTOLOGY

THE body of a multicellular organism is composed of a very large number of cells, most of which contain a nucleus in which the genetic, hereditable material of the cell is found. The nuclei of all cells contain the same amount of genetic material. This can be shown by spectrophotometric measurements, and, if the cell can be induced to divide and preparations of the metaphase chromosomes can be made, it is found that the chromosome number and pattern for each of the cells of the body are the same. It is, indeed, part of the central concept of genetics that each cell nucleus contains all the hereditable material necessary for the full expression of the form and function of the individual. Hybridization experiments, in which cell nuclei from two species are incorporated into the cytoplasm of one cell, show that genetic material capable of coding for the proteins of many enzymes is present in a single somatic cell nucleus. Examination of cells in the living body and in histological and cytological preparations shows, however, that there is a wide range of form and function. Some cells are small and have little cytoplasm, others, such as the anterior horn cells of the spinal cord or the Betz cells of the cerebral cortex, have cytoplasmic processes up to a metre in length. The functions of cells differ widely; striated muscle cells have the capacity to contract in response to nervous stimuli, squamous epithelial cells form a protective keratin coat, intestinal mucosal cells secrete mucin and a series of digestive enzymes, and the cells of the endocrine organs elaborate hormones which are released into the circulation and, in turn, control the activity of other cells.

This wide diversity of cytoplasmic form and of physiological function is highly ordered. We do not find bone-cells in the skin epidermis or squamous epithelium lining the colon. We do find nerve-cells connected to motor end-plates which, in turn, are applied to striated muscle cells, the various epithelia of the hollow viscera are surrounded by supporting tissues which, themselves, are invested by a functioning coat of unstriated muscle. The pattern for this complex organization which determines both the form and function of cells and their relative spatial disposition is included in the genetic material of the zygote, the first cell of the individual formed by the fusion of the maternal ovum and the paternal spermatozoa, and is expressed through the complex sequence of changes during development which we consider under the term 'embryology'.

NORMAL DEVELOPMENT

Normal development is a sequential process. In the earliest stages of embryonic life the embryo consists of a ball of indistinguishable cells and division of this group of cells into two gives rise to two separate individuals, monozygotic twins. As the ball of cells increases in size, the cells at the centre, which are surrounded by the cells at the periphery, have a different environment from those at the external surface and begin to grow differently; eventually fluid collects and a hollow sphere, the blastocyst, is formed. The crucial change is the development of craniocaudal orientation which begins at this stage. One group of cells, called the 'primary organizer' or 'Henson's node', produces substances which affect the adjacent cells and introduce a direction of growth. In some animals this orientation is mediated by differences in the cytoplasm of the ovum at its two poles. Once the sequence has been started, each group of cells interacts with its neighbours and differentiation begins. At first the embryo forms a disk of two-cell layers one of which, the ectoderm, is to form the integumentary tissues and the central nervous system, while the other, the endoderm, is to form the lining of the alimentary tract and its related tubular viscera, and also most of the solid glandular organs. The third germ layer, the mesoderm, is formed of cells which grow between the two layers of the embryonic disk and this layer gives origin to the supporting tissues of the body, and also the excretory and reproductive organs. Detailed organization, in response to the action of evoking and inducing substances, continues during embryonic life. For example, the mesodermal tissue adjacent to bronchial epithelium becomes differentiated into cartilage and the anlage of a joint shows a sequence of synovium, cartilage, and bone. Further development continues during extra-embryonic life; the kidney at birth often contains primitive tubules and glomeruli and the reproductive organs undergo changes in structure and functional capacity in response to the hormonal changes of puberty, pregnancy, and the menopause.

The changes in form and function of cells during embryonic life are mediated by changes in genetic capacity. Once a cell is committed to being a squamous epithelial cell, it will for the most part breed true, both in its natural situation and also if it is transplanted elsewhere in the body. This implies that there are controlling changes in the genetic material of the cell which are in turn hereditable. The mechanisms of these changes are by no means understood, but a useful analogy is the 'book model'. The genetic material can be compared to a set of instructions contained in a series of three books. At the zygote stage and in the earliest phases of embryonic life, the full set of instructions is available. As the cells become committed to one of the three germ layers, two of the books are sealed and only the third is available. Further commitment, to skin or central nervous tissue, to bone or kidney, to colonic mucosa or pancreas, involves selection of a chapter and sealing of the rest of the books. Final differentiation, for example as a striated muscle cell, involves selection of a paragraph and a blocking of the rest of the chapter. Such blocking may be due to chemical combination of histones, proteins found only in association with chromosomal material, with the DNA bases; it may be due to cross-linking of the DNA bases; or it may be due to the activity of specialized repressor genes. The level of blocking also varies; once commitment to a germ layer takes place, the blocking is complete. At levels further along the path of differentiation blocking is less complete and redifferentiation in a different but allied form may be possible. There are also some metabolic functions common to all cells which might be imagined to be included as an introduction which remain freely available, and there is a supplement concerned with the process of cell division which is available to many cells but not to all. The red blood-cells have no nucleus and cannot divide, the cells of striated muscle and the nerve-cells of the central nervous system similarly are incapable of cell division.

METAPLASIA

The mode of differentiation is not immutable. The cells of many tissues retain the capacity for differentiation in more than one way in response to external stimuli. The bronchial mucosa normally consists of glandular cells equipped with cilia and arranged in a pattern termed 'pseudostratified'; the bronchial lining of a patient suffering from chronic bronchitis, however, or that of a cigarette smoker, consists of a protective squamous epithelium. These changes, termed 'metaplasia', can occur in epithelial or in connective tissues and represent the fraction of the genome in which blocking is incomplete and unblocking is easily achieved. It is as though a page can easily be turned while a separate chapter is out of reach.

In most tissues it is probable that the fully differentiated cells which are exercising the functions of the tissue are normally incapable of cell division, and that there are stem cells, found, for example, in the basal area of squamous epithelium and in the depths of the intestinal crypts or as the myeloblasts and erythroblasts of the bone-marrow, which have the potential for differentiation but retain the capacity for cell division. Any metabolic process, whether it be the excretion of enzymes, the secretion of hormones, or the formation of bone matrix or keratinized squames, requires energy and similarly the process of cell division is energy consuming. The physical size of a cell sets a limit to the amount of energy which can be utilized and hence a limit to the range of metabolic processes which can be carried out. It has been estimated that cell division requires at least one-third of the available energy which a cell can use.

DIFFERENTIATION IN TUMOURS

The foregoing discussion of normal development and normal function is very relevant to the study of neoplastic growth and development. Most tumour cells show some evidence of differentiation; the cytoplasm of the cells shows the structure, or an approximation to the structure, of the cells from which it takes origin. This is reflected in the nomenclature of tumours (CHAPTER II). We distinguish on histological grounds between carcinoma, the tumour of epithelial cells, and sarcoma, the tumour of connective-tissue cells. Within these groups we recognize squamous-cell carcinoma and adenocarcinoma; we identify osteosarcoma, fibrosarcoma, liposarcoma, and so on. These differences between tumour cells reflect the degree and type of blocking of the cells from which they take origin. When a cell becomes neoplastic the capacity to multiply is freed from the normal mechanisms of control, but some or all of the blocking of genetic material which is characteristic of the normal cell from which it arises remains, and the origin can be identified. This persistent histological appearance is often even more subtle than is indicated by the descriptive terms given to tumour types. In many instances histological examination of a secondary deposit of tumour enables the pathologist to give an intelligent guess at the site of origin of the primary lesion. This is partly based on a knowledge of the types of tumour which commonly occur in various situations and also on recognition of evidence of differentiation in the cells.

I suggested above that the capacity of a cell for function is limited by the amount of energy available to it and that the process of cell division requires a substantial fraction of the available energy resources of the cell. This leads to two factors of importance in the field of oncology. First, if, as is probable, the fully differentiated cell is committed to function rather than to reproduction, the frequency of tumours of various tissues and various cell types will depend on the degree of differentiation and on the presence of stem cells. The carcinomata arise from epithelial cells; these for the most part are concerned with protection of the body from the environment or with the secretion of substances on to the surface of the body and into the body cavities. In both cases there is a high rate of cell loss, the superficial cells of a squamous epithelium are continually being lost to the surface and are being replaced by fresh cells from the basal layers. Similarly the cells of the gastro-intestinal mucosa are continually being lost into the contents of the digestive tract and are being replaced by the multiplying cells of the deeper parts of the crypts. Almost the whole of the lining membrane of the uterus is lost monthly at menstruation and is replaced by growth from the few remaining basal glands. Tumours of the squamous epithelia and of the glandular epithelia of these organs are common. In contrast the striated cells of the voluntary muscles and the nerve-cells of the central and peripheral nervous system are not lost in large numbers and are not replaced if they are lost. Some of the manifestations of senescence has been said to be due to the death of nerve-cells without subsequent replacement. Tumours of these cells are exceedingly rare. Similarly the red blood-cell represents the ultimate in differentiation. It consists only of a sac full of respiratory protein and has no nucleus and therefore no reproductive capacity. A tumour of red cells, 'erythrocytoma', is impossible.

Secondly, the apportionment of energy between differentiation and reproduction, the rapidly multiplying cell being less capable of showing differentiative activity, is the basis for the rule that the less well-differentiated tumour is the one with greater malignant potential. This observation is used in the histological grading of tumours which can form a useful adjunct to the diagnostic process, to establishing a prognosis and to the management of the patient. It may be considered that the greater the evidence of differentiation in the cells of a tumour, the greater the proportion of the energy-consuming activity of the tumour is diverted to functional activity, while the more the activity of the tumour cells is directed to reproduction the less available energy is left for somatic function. The grading of tumours which may be expected on this theoretical basis is confirmed by clinicopathological observations; a well-differentiated squamous-cell carcinoma of the lung is, if it is accessible to surgery, more likely to be cured by excision than is a lung tumour composed of small cells without evidence of differentiation of the cells either into a squamous or a glandular form.

MIXED TUMOURS

The hypothesis of sequential differentiation and of blocking of the genetic material must also be capable of explaining the finding of tumours of mixed cellular type. The most extreme form of mixture of cell types is seen in the teratomata which are, for other reasons, peculiar tumours outside the usual pattern, and these are discussed separately in CHAPTER XV. The majority of mixed tumours contain elements of connective-tissue origin which are closely related; cartilage and bone are seen together in the body and as tumours in the osteochondromata, fibrous tissue is seen adjacent to small blood-vessels in the normal tissues and in the angiofibromata. In these cases and in such epithelial tumours as lung cancer where both squamous and glandular elements may coexist, and in bladder cancer where the tumour may contain squamous, transitional, and glandular epithelium, it may be suggested that a potential differentiative capacity exists, and that a small degree of unblocking only is required. In other cases of apparently mixed tumours the connective-tissue element may represent metaplastic change in the cells of the stroma surrounding epithelial neoplastic cells. In mixed salivary tumours the presence of extracellular mucin from the cells of the salivary epithelium may induce a cartilaginous appearance in the cells of the stroma (*Fig.* 5), and areas of bone are sometimes seen in the connective tissue adjacent to cancer of the breast or to metastatic deposits from cancer of the bladder.

A third mode of origin of mixed tumours is seen in the hamartomata, lesions in which there is overgrowth of both epithelial and connective tissues in a way resembling the association of these structures in the normal body. Such a lesion is the cartilaginous hamartoma of the bronchus which consists of a mass of cartilage surrounding cystic spaces and ducts lined by epithelium of bronchial type. Some of these lesions are under hormonal control; for example, the fibro-adenoma of the breast, seen usually in the first half of reproductive life, in which both glandular and fibrous elements show comparable overgrowth. Other lesions of this type have a genetic basis; in tuberose sclerosis, determined by a dominant gene, there is overgrowth of glial tissues in the brain, sebaceous glands in the skin, fibrous tissue in the gums, and an admixture of smooth muscle, fat, and blood-vessels in the kidney and liver. The effect of this gene appears to be, by some mechanism which is quite unknown, to release blocks of cells from the normal control mechanisms within the organs.

The final type of mixed tumour is more complex in its histology and less easy to interpret. This is the mixed mesodermal tumour seen most often in the uterine cavity, but also very occasionally elsewhere, in which there is a conglomeration of different connective-tissue elements, bone cartilage, fat, smooth and striated muscle, and fibrous tissue being massed together without apparent order (*Fig.* 6). In the case of the uterine neoplasm, elements of undoubted epithelial form are also seen. These tumours represent in their differentiation an unblocking of all the genes responsible for the expression of connective-tissue differentiation and in different parts of the tumour a reordering of differentiation in different ways. The presence of the epithelial element in mixed mesodermal tumour of the uterus, which is probably the only true carcinosarcoma, reminds us that the epithelial lining of the uterine cavity, which is derived from the Müllerian ducts, is of mesodermal origin and is neither ectodermal nor endodermal.

ABERRANT DIFFERENTIATION

Aberrant differentiation, the development in tumour cells of manifestations of differentiation which was not present in the cells of origin, is also sometimes seen when release of genetic blocking occurs. In some cases the evidence for abnormal differentiation is anatomical. Osteosarcomata have been seen in the soft tissues of the muscles and fascia in the lung, and in the supporting tissues of the breast. In other cases the evidence of abnormal function is chemical, hormones are produced by the cells of tumours of apparently non-endocrine nature. A number of examples of small-cell tumour of the lung have been described in which an excessive activity of one or more hormones has been detected. Most such hormonal activity depends on the production and release of a single protein substance and on the basis of the template of a single sequence of DNA bases and can therefore be regarded as a relatively small abnormal unblocking of genetic material.

CHAPTER VI

THE PRECANCEROUS STATE: CARCINOMA-IN-SITU

It has been recognized for very many years that lesions may be found in the human body which, in time, will develop malignant propensities and evolve into neoplasms having all the characteristics of carcinomata and sarcomata, including metastasis and the death of the patient. Some of these conditions are determined by the action of abnormal dominant genes which result in the production of benign tumour-like lesions such as the multiple polyps of polyposis coli, the hamartomata of tuberose sclerosis, or the cartilage-capped exostoses of diaphysial aclasis, and the development of malignant change is related to the greatly increased number of cells available for neoplastic transformation and to the aberrant control mechanisms in these conditions. These lesions, together with xeroderma pigmentosa in which the basic lesion is a defect in the repair mechanism of DNA in the cell nuclei, are discussed in CHAPTER X. In such conditions the cells are transformed by environmental factors which, less often, cause malignant transformation of the normal cells of the parts affected. It is noteworthy in this connexion that the colonic polyps frequently undergo malignant change while the hamartomatous small intestinal polyps of the Peutz-Jegher syndrome rarely do so, a difference corresponding to the frequency of carcinoma in the intact colon and the rarity of such tumours in the small intestine.

There remains a group of conditions in which a lesion usually classified as benign frequently undergoes malignant change. Some of these lesions form recognizable clinical entities in which a diagnosis can be made by inspection of the lesion. Queyrat's erythroplasia is manifest as shiny or velvety red plaques in the epithelium of the glans penis or in the inner surface of the prepuce. Histologically there is seen to be disorderly proliferation of the squamous cells of the epithelium, often with large, clear, swollen cells in groups and clusters. Bowen's disease of the skin is a similar lesion which may occur anywhere on the surface of the body. Initially the lesions, which may be multicentric, form scaly red areas which later develop into nodules which may be crusted or eroded. The histological changes are again those of disorderly epithelial proliferation without invasion through the basement

THE PRECANCEROUS STATE: CARCINOMA-IN-SITU

membrane. The third eponymous precancerous lesion is Paget's disease of the nipple, which is a localized red granular lesion resembling eczema which may later become ulcerated. There is disorderly epithelial proliferation and in the epithelium there are characteristic 'Paget cells' which are large, oval or elongated cells with a round or oval nucleus and clear or finely granular cytoplasm. The lesion may extend down the ducts of the nipple or may extend outwards from abnormal cells in the mammary acini and is associated sooner or later with adenocarcinoma of the breast.

A similar status may be accorded to leucoplakia, a clinical entity comprising a white lesion of a usually moist squamous epithelium especially of the mouth or of the vulva.

A second clinically identifiable form of precancerous lesion is seen in benign tumours which frequently become malignant. The three commonest manifestations of this phenomenon are papilloma of the bladder, intraduct carcinoma of the breast, and senile keratosis of the skin. In all three cases the lesion consists of cells not very far removed histologically from the normal and confined within a small space. The proliferating transitional cells of the bladder papilloma are separated from the fibrous stroma of the polypoid lesion and do not show invasion. The neoplastic cells of intraduct carcinoma of the breast fill, and may expand, the duct, but do not extend into the surrounding tissues, and the proliferating squamous cells of the wart-like lesion of senile keratosis are confined by the basement membrane of the skin. These three lesions are, however, regarded as intrinsically neoplastic and if they are left alone or are removed incompletely the development of invasive properties is very likely.

Finally, there is a group of lesions which is not apparent on clinical examination and in which the diagnosis is made on the basis of histological or cytological examination of tissue or cells removed for some other reason or in the course of a screening procedure. The major members of this group are carcinoma-in-situ of the uterine cervix, the so-called 'latent' carcinoma of the prostate, and the condition of adenoma malignum in otherwise benign polyps of the colon. Carcinoma-in-situ of the cervix is detectable by histological examination of cells from the surface of the cervical epithelium, removed by gentle scraping of the cervical os, or by collection of cells desquamated into the vaginal fluid. The ease of collection of such specimens has led to a great deal of attention being focused on this condition. The macroscopic appearance of the cervix is usually either normal or it shows the changes of chronic cervicitis which are very frequent in women who have borne children. On histological examination there is the same type of disorderly cell proliferation which is seen in the lesions mentioned above. The major point of histological identification is that the usual progression of cell types in an organized squamous epithelium is lost. Normally there is a basal layer of cubical or columnar cells arranged with their long axes perpendicular to the basement membrane and to the surface. These are the cells which are capable of multiplication and from which the upper layers are formed; as the cells pass from the basal layer to the surface to replace those which are lost by desquamation they change shape and become more flattened and, in the superficial layers, begin to form keratin. In carcinoma-in-situ this orderly progression is lost, dividing cells may be seen at any level in the epithelium and keratinization may be apparent in the deeper zones (*Fig.* 7). A similar histological abnormality may be seen in the cells of squamous epithelium adjacent to any squamous carcinoma and is a well-defined feature of the bronchial mucosa which has undergone squamous metaplasia and has developed squamous carcinoma. Similar lesions are seen in the larynx, and, less often, in the skin. These sites are less accessible to collection of cells for cytological examination and it is unusual for carcinoma-in-situ to be diagnosed in the absence of a clinically evident squamous-celled carcinoma.

Latent carcinoma of the prostate is a condition which has been recognized by the histological examination of sections of prostates removed at autopsy or because of benign prostatic hyperplasia. The frequency of this lesion is extremely high. In some series of cases it has been reported that more than 80 per cent of men over the age of 80 years have such changes in their prostate glands. From the point of view of the histologist it is much more difficult to separate this lesion from classic clinical carcinoma of the prostate.

In the third member of this group, adenoma malignum arising in colonic polyps (*Fig.* 8), the histological distinction is made on the basis of loss of differentiation. The cells of the colonic polyp generally resemble closely the cells of the colonic mucosa and show evidence of mucus secretion and retention. The lesion of adenoma malignum is characterized by loss of the capacity to produce mucin, the cytoplasm is eosinophilic rather than vacuolated, the nucleus is usually a little larger, and the chromatin is less densely compacted.

It is this last group of precancerous lesions which poses the greatest problems in the field of general tumour pathology. Malignant transformation of a benign tumour, whether due to genetic processes or occurring apparently spontaneously, is easy to interpret in accordance with a theory of tumour development involving a succession of stages (CHAPTER VIII) and the lesions which can be detected and diagnosed clinically require treatment on their own merits. The likely clinical course of the diseases is well known and appropriate measures of therapy or of surveillance can be instituted. For example, in the case of polyposis coli it is now accepted that most of the colon should be removed, leaving the rectum with its sphincters, as soon as the diagnosis is established, thereby preventing the certain development of carcinoma. The polyps in the small remaining segment are kept under surveillance by regular sigmoidoscopy. Similarly if Paget's disease of the nipple is identified, the breast is removed. However, when the diagnosis rests on histological criteria only, and especially when cytological screening procedures are possible, the clinicopathological problem becomes more difficult.

Both carcinoma and carcinoma-in-situ are disease entities, that is to say each can be defined quite rigorously and there is a substantial body of agreement over the diagnosis of each. The difficulty which arises is that they are disease entities of different types. The concept of malignant disease in general and of carcinomata in particular is of a dynamic clinical condition which has a predictable course. A malignant tumour will, if left alone, spread and metastasize and will eventually cause the death of the patient. The other criteria which are used in diagnosis, and especially the histological criteria, are subordinate to this clinical concept. When the histologist examines a section of tissue and reports carcinoma or sarcoma he is making a correlation between the histological appearance which he sees and the clinical course of patients who have had similar histological lesions. He is in effect saying, 'This lesion is similar to other lesions which have spread and caused death.' The basis even of the histological report is therefore clinical. In the case of carcinoma-in-situ of the cervix and of latent carcinoma of the prostate, the basis of the entity is different. In these conditions the static histological appearance of the lesion is the basic criterion on which the concept is based. There are differences in the type and arrangement of the tissue cells which resemble, but are not identical with, those of fully established malignancy and usually represent an intermediate stage. Once it is appreciated that these conditions are histological entities rather than clinical entities, it follows that study to establish the clinical connotation to be applied to these terms is required. This is of the greatest importance because if this correlation is not carried out errors in management are liable to occur. In particular, two conceptual errors have crept into both surgical and pathological usage. These may be summarized in the form of two statements: 'All carcinomata pass through a period of in-situ-carcinoma', 'In-situ-carcinomata are a stage in the development of carcinoma and should be treated vigorously'.

These two statements follow from a ready acceptance of the histological concept of in-situ-carcinoma and a transfer of the term carcinoma to its clinical connotation. The first statement is ultimately true in that in the earliest stages of malignant transformation the tumour consists of a very few cells, possibly only one cell which is still situated in a normal histological locus. The statement, however, carries the implication that this early stage can be recognized and that if it can be detected the tumour could be eradicated at this stage. It is probable that in many tumours the stage which could be considered 'in situ' is very short and that the capacity to invade the surrounding tissues is a character which the malignant cells develop very early so that even when the lesion is microscopic in size and amounts to only a few tens of cells, some of these have invaded and even passed away from the primary site in the bloodstream or lymphatics. It is certainly true that in most tumours there is no prolonged stage of 'in situ' neoplasm which, if detected, would provide an opportunity for certain cure. This is true even in the cervix, the type situation of in-situ-carcinoma, where invasive lesions have been seen only a few months after cytological examination has been negative.

The second statement is somewhat suspect. The only way in which one could know with certainty that the lesion of in-situ-carcinoma invariably progresses to carcinoma would be to leave patients with this lesion and observe progress. This has been done in the case of a small series of carcinoma-in-situ of the cervix and it has been found that less than half developed overt carcinoma within an observation period of 10 years. This type of clinical observation is difficult for several reasons. First, the use of the term 'carcinoma', with its clinical connotations, brings problems of the ethics of clinical experimentation; is it ethically right to leave such patients without treatment? Secondly, there is the biological equivalent of Heisenberg's Principle of Uncertainty. In order to establish the diagnosis of carcinoma-in-situ it is necessary to examine the lesion histologically. To do this it must be removed, and it could be argued that, in those patients who do not go on to develop overt carcinoma, the lesion was removed completely at the biopsy. Conversely, it could be argued that in those patients who do go on to develop carcinoma there was a small carcinoma left behind in the material not taken for biopsy. An additional problem is posed by the query of how long a period of development should be expected. A lesion which takes 30 years to progress from an in-situ stage to frank malignancy is unlikely to be of clinical significance in a patient of 80. Some epidemiological studies have been carried out in the case of carcinoma-in-situ of the cervix, which is sufficiently common for data susceptible of analysis to be available, and it appears probable that at least half the lesions of in-situ-carcinoma in this organ do not progress to overt carcinoma but rather regress perhaps as a consequence of immune reaction.

The difficulty of clinicohistological correlation is even more apparent in the case of latent carcinoma of the prostate. On the one hand, it is stated by expert and experienced histologists that this lesion is present in the majority of men over the age of 75 years. On the other hand, clinical and pathological experience shows that carcinoma of the prostate is the cause of death in only a small proportion of men even at the most advanced ages. The impasse is resolved if it is recognized that the lesion of latent carcinoma observed by the histologist is a benign condition which usually remains so during the life span of the patient but which may undergo further changes which confer upon it a malignant potential. Acceptance of this concept makes the management of patients in whom this condition is recognized after prostatectomy much easier. The operation can be regarded as curative and an expectant attitude adopted rather than the use of hormones or further surgical procedures.

The problems of precancerous states of whatever type become easier to understand and the clinical management of patients in whom these conditions are seen becomes more reasonable if the overriding importance of the clinical correlation with the histological findings is appreciated, and if it is recognized that in many of these conditions full neoplastic development requires further changes in the cells mediated by some environmental agent. In some cases, such as polyposis coli and Paget's disease of the nipple, progression to carcinoma is almost inevitable, and radical therapy is required. In other cases, such as diaphysial aclasis and latent carcinoma of the prostate, surveillance is the mode of management of choice. In yet others, local excision of a lesion, such as a patch of leucoplakia, or a solitary rectal polyp, will suffice. It has been interesting to note over the years how the recommended surgical approach to in-situ-carcinoma of the cervix has progressed from hysterectomy through amputation of the cervix, to a deep cone biopsy followed by observation as the clinical connotation of the lesion has become more apparent.

CHAPTER VII
PROGRESSION AND REGRESSION

THE contrasting phenomena of progression and regression are of great importance in an understanding of the nature of malignant disease and in applying a knowledge of the pathological processes to a rational method of treatment and management. Progression is a process in which the character of a tumour changes during its life in such a way that the clinical course is worsened, the tumour grows more rapidly or becomes better able to spread locally, and to metastasize. Regression is the opposite process, in which the character of the tumour as seen in the living patient changes in a way which is beneficial to the patient. Either it becomes more readily susceptible to treatment or it even disappears altogether.

PROGRESSION

If biopsies are made of a tumour at intervals during its life cycle, either as repeated samples of a tumour which remains in situ and is regarded as unsuitable for treatment, or if samples are taken from a tumour at the time of excision and later from recurrent growths, it will often be found that the histological appearance changes. The change in appearance is most often in the direction of increasing malignancy. The histological appearance corresponds in successive biopsies to that seen in tumours of increasingly rapid growth and increasing liability to metastasize. The degree of expression of the differentiative potentiality of the cells decreases; in an initial biopsy there may be fully formed squamous epithelium with keratinization and the formation of epithelial pearls; in a later biopsy the squamous origin of the lesion may be recognizable by the pattern of cell shapes in a gradient away from the stroma and the blood-supply, but keratinization, the full expression of a squamous nature, is absent; in a third biopsy even these indications of squamous differentiation may be lost and the lesion may consist of small polygonal cells without any evidence of specific differentiation (*Figs.* 9, 10). *Pari passu* with these changes in differentiation come changes in the regularity of cell size and shape; in the later biopsies large and small, regular and irregular cells are intermingled and evidence of an increase in multiplicative potential is given by an increase in the proportion of cells showing the various stages of mitosis.

When multiple sections are taken from various parts of a large tumour a similar variation in histological structure, this time distributed in space rather than in time, is often seen, and it is a tacit acceptance of the principle of progression that a report on such a tumour gives a grading according to the least well-differentiated part (*Figs.* 11, 12). A large brain tumour may show areas of well-defined oligodendroglia with other areas of astrocytoma and still other areas in which the appearance is that of glioblastoma multiforme: from the point of view of the patient and of the surgeon the tumour is regarded as being of the most malignant type, a conclusion later to be borne out by the clinical course.

More recently it has been possible to prepare tumour cells in such a way that analysis of the chromosomes is possible and serial karyotype analyses of the cells of leukaemias have shown a similar progression in departure from the normal pattern of chromosome constitution. At an early stage in the disease the chromosome pattern is little different from the normal; later cells with grossly abnormal chromosome patterns come to dominate the picture.

Finally, a study of the histological appearance of metastatic deposits may show evidence of this phenomenon. If a number of sections are taken from various parts of a large tumour a range of histological appearances may be seen. Histological examination of the secondary deposits in lymph-nodes or other organs will show the deposits to correspond in histological features to the less well-differentiated, the more malignant, parts of the primary tumour.

This phenomenon is readily understandable if the tumour is regarded as a population of cells which take origin from the cells of the host, but which are independent of the host, and can react by adaptive changes to changes in the environment. A clinical example of this is seen in the case of acute leukaemia where a patient commonly shows a remission when treated with a chemotherapeutic agent, for example a corticosteroid or a folic acid antagonist, but when on maintenance therapy a relapse occurs, and the lesion is thereafter not sensitive to the initial drug. One remission per drug is a rough but fairly accurate guide. The population of tumour cells eventually comes to number many hundreds and thousands of millions and will come to be dominated by those cells best able to adapt to the environment in which they find themselves and best able to multiply and to spread to other environments within the body. The cells which survive are those which are, within the ecological niche, the fittest. The normal cells of the body are subject to a wide variety of controls which establish the constancy of form and function which is a characteristic of the multicellular organism. Tumour cells, on the other hand, are freed from many of these restraints and are able to survive and to multiply after changes in their character which in a somatic cell would lead to destruction by the controlling agencies. In the case of a multicellular organism most changes induced by mutation are deleterious because they do not fit into the complex pattern of activities necessary for the growth and function of a complicated entity. In the case of a clone of tumour cells, each of which may be regarded as a separate individual from the evolutionary point of view, deleterious changes can and do occur. It is probable that the monstrous giant cells with multilobed irregular nuclei seen in some tumours are examples of deleterious change in cells and that such cells are incapable of mitosis and have reached the end of an evolutionary road. Such cells form only a small proportion of the cells of a tumour and in time are replaced by others better able to multiply and to survive.

As the clinician and the pathologist look at the phenomenon of progression it often appears to be a stepwise process. Areas of tumour are seen of one or another histological type. A patient has relatively clearly defined remissions and relapses. To some extent this is correct, because we can only observe these changes in the character of tumour cells which are so advantageous as to produce large changes in biological character, or in histological appearance. These correspond to the large changes in flora and fauna which have been observed as living things have evolved in the history of the world, but, like the changes in animals and in plants, are the large-scale expression of a multitude of small-scale changes.

The phenomenon of progression is discussed here in relation to the changes which occur in a developed malignant neoplasm. This, I think, is a correct view to take as it is only at the stage of established malignancy that the cells of the tumour can be regarded as a separate colony of cells capable of change and of evolutionary adaptation. Serial changes such as the progress from carcinoma-in-situ to invasive carcinoma or from colonic polyp through adenoma malignum to invasive carcinoma and the transformation from benign to malignant represent changes in the cells of the body which are still under the control of the homeostatic mechanism. The changes which lead to release from normal control appear to be more closely defined than those which occur in a developed tumour and will be discussed with a consideration of the problems of oncogenesis in CHAPTER VIII.

The concept of progression has direct clinical significance. The likelihood of changes in the cells of a tumour is a very strong indication for the earliest possible treatment and the detectable differences within the substance of a single mass of tumour tissue may guide those responsible for the postoperative management of the patient. Furthermore, the possibility of adaptation to a therapeutic régime makes it necessary to continue investigations designed to improve on the methods of treatment already available and to devise new methods.

REGRESSION

Regression, spontaneous disappearance of a tumour, or a spontaneous change in the character of a tumour, is a much less common clinical

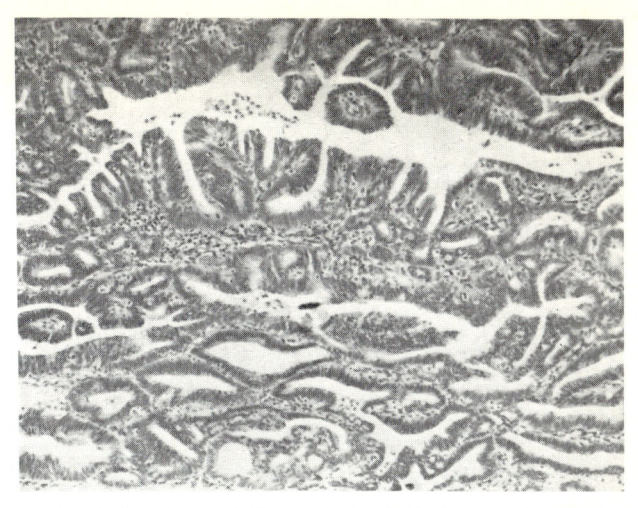

Fig. 1.—Atypical endometrial hyperplasia. This is an endometrial curetting showing distortion and crowding of the glands. The appearance is highly atypical but does not conform to the usual criteria of malignancy. The uterus was removed and no invasive tumour was found. (× 80.)

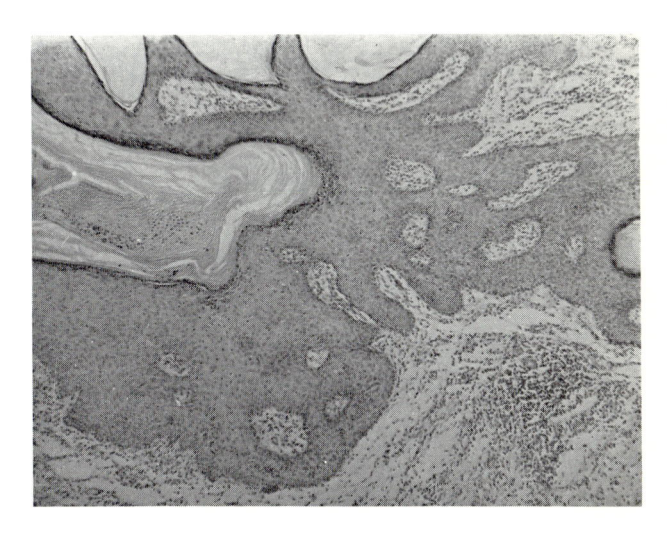

Fig. 2.—Squamous-cell papilloma. A benign tumour of skin. There is excessive growth but no invasion has occurred and the differentiative function of the skin, formation of keratin, is retained. (× 50.)

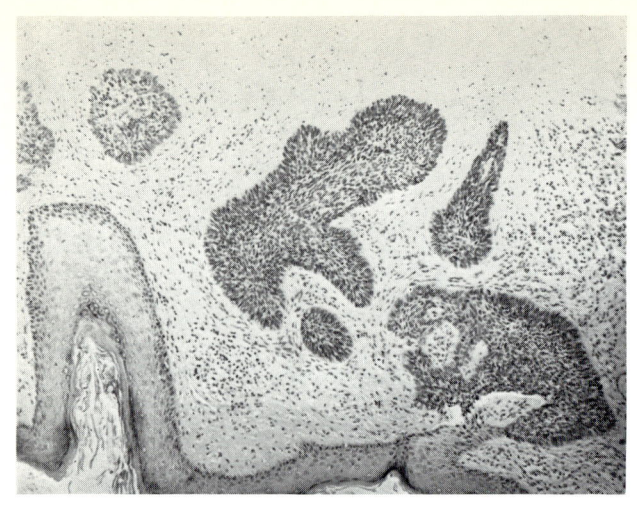

Fig. 3.—Basal-cell carcinoma. A second skin tumour in which the neoplastic process involves the deeper cells of the epidermis which invade the dermis but remain in coherent groups. While this type of tumour has an invasive propensity it is unlikely to metastasize. (× 64.)

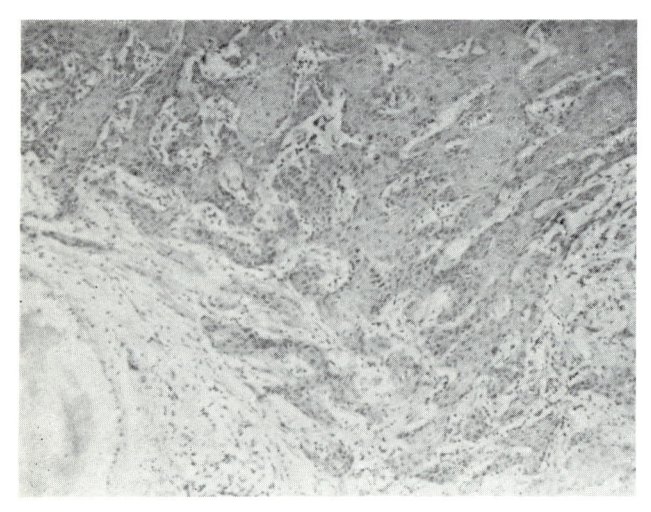

Fig. 4.—Squamous-cell carcinoma. The malignant tumour of skin and of other squamous epithelia. There is still a tendency to produce keratinized squames but invasion and metastasis by the lymphatics is common. (× 80.)

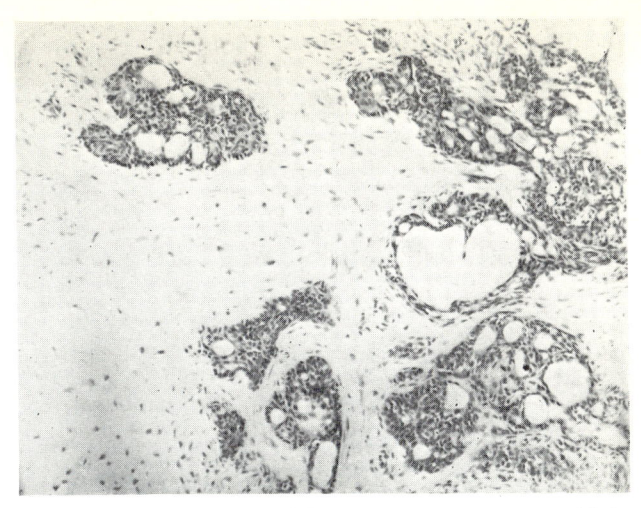

Fig. 5.—Mixed salivary tumour. The cartilaginous appearance of the stroma of this epithelial tumour is probably due to inductive influences from the neoplastic cells. This contrasts with the truly mixed tumour (*Fig.* 6). (×80.)

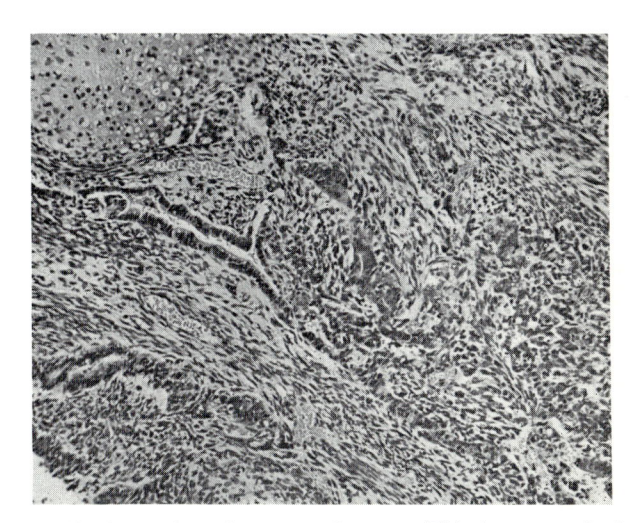

Fig. 6.—Mixed mesodermal tumour of uterus. This is a true mixed tumour arising in the endometrium which is wholly of mesodermal origin. The connective tissue and cartilage are neoplastic as is the epithelial tissue. (×80.)

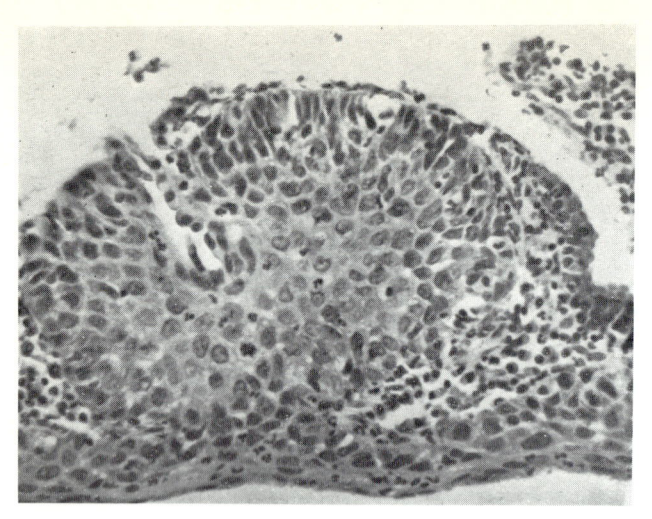

Fig. 7.—Carcinoma-in-situ of cervix. Neoplastic change has occurred in the cells which are still confined to the normal situation of cervical epithelium. There is distortion of the pattern of differentiation but no invasion is seen. Regression of this lesion can occur. (× 256.)

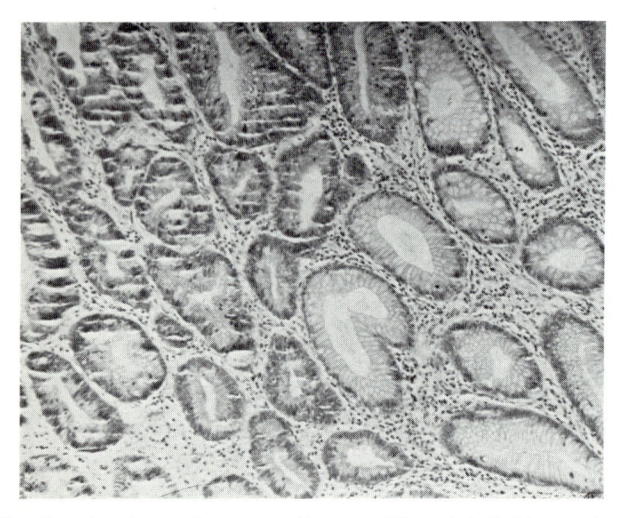

Fig. 8.—Rectal polyp—adenoma malignum. The acini of this rectal polyp are of two types. Some resemble normal colonic epithelia closely and in the others there is less mucin production and the cell nuclei are dense and closely packed. Local excision of this lesion is a satisfactory form of treatment. (× 80.)

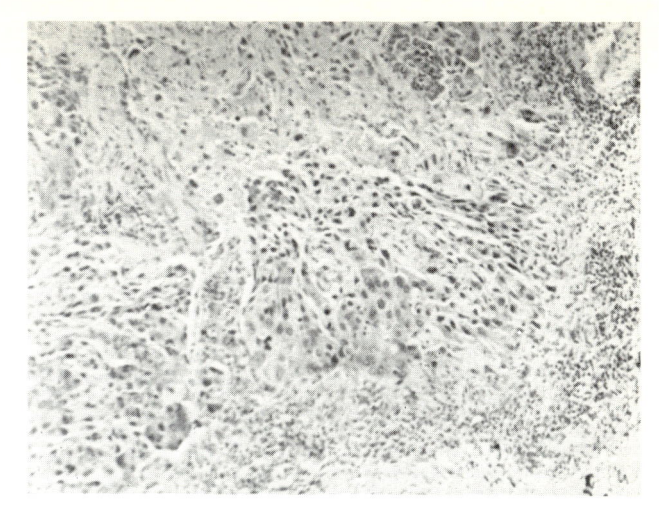

Fig. 9.—Poorly differentiated squamous-cell carcinoma of lung. (× 80.)

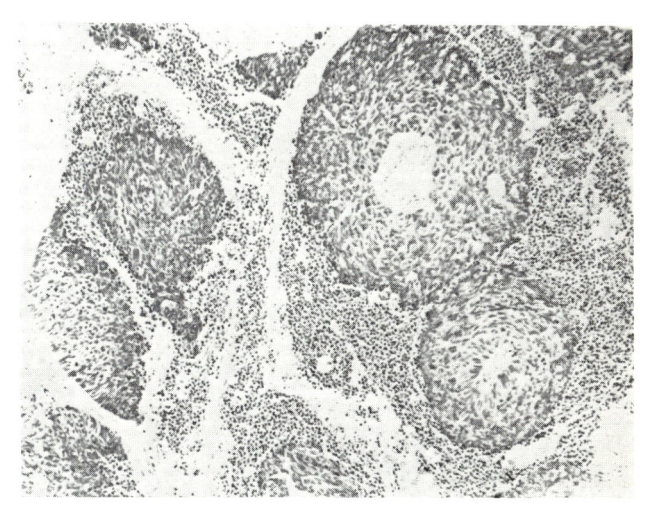

Fig. 10.—Undifferentiated carcinoma of lung. These two photomicrographs are taken from a lung tumour and an invaded lymph-node respectively. They illustrate the difference in histological appearance between the primary tumour and a metastasis and show the progression of histological form which may occur. (× 80.)

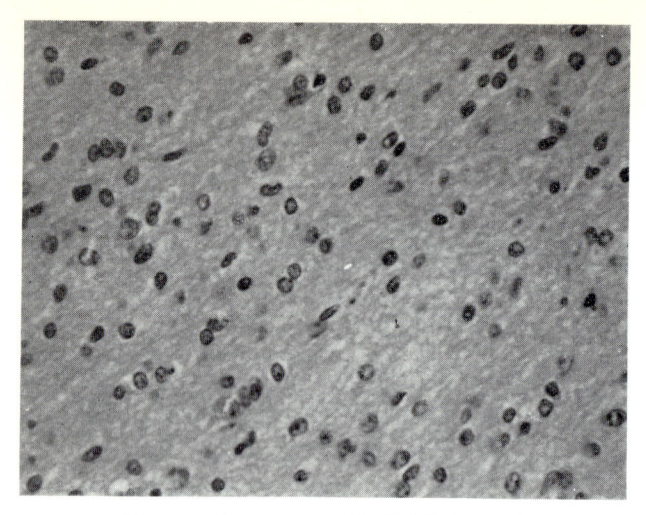

Fig. 11.—Astrocytoma, Grade II. (× 320.)

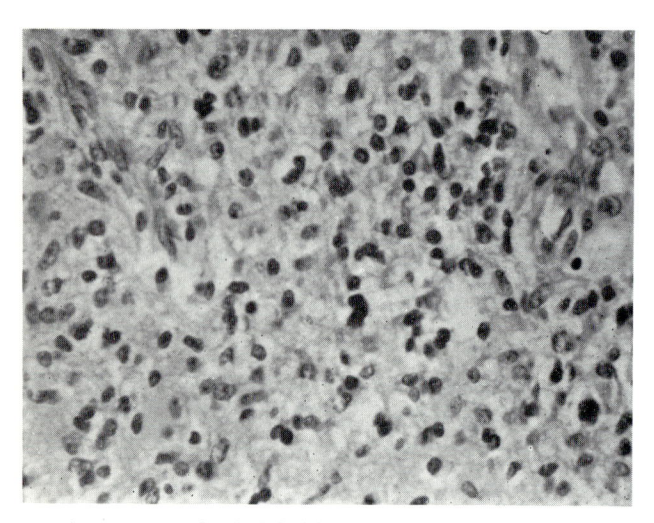

Fig. 12.—Astrocytoma, Grade IV. Two photomicrographs taken from a single section of a brain tumour. One shows a less cellular lesion comprising cells of uniform size and shape, while in the other field there is variation in cell size and shape. The tumour may be expected to behave clinically as a rapidly progressive neoplasm of Grade IV. (× 320.)

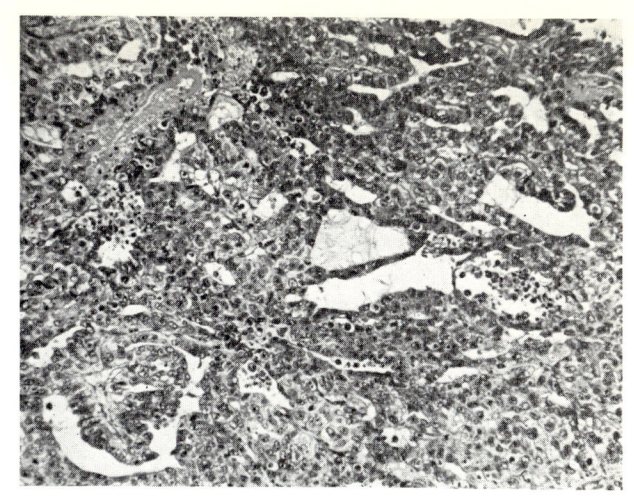

Fig. 13.—Embryonal carcinoma of testis. A malignant epithelial teratoma of the testis. The cells are of epithelial form and are arranged in a roughly acinar pattern. Organoid differentiation is not seen. (×92.)

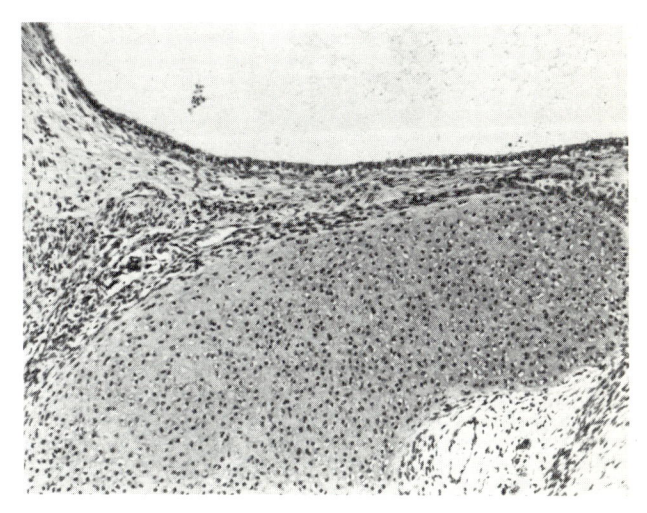

Fig. 14.—Respiratory organoid development in a teratoma. The epithelium in this part of the tumour is columnar and ciliated and is closely related to muscle tissue and a block of cartilage in a manner normally seen in the bronchi. (×80.)

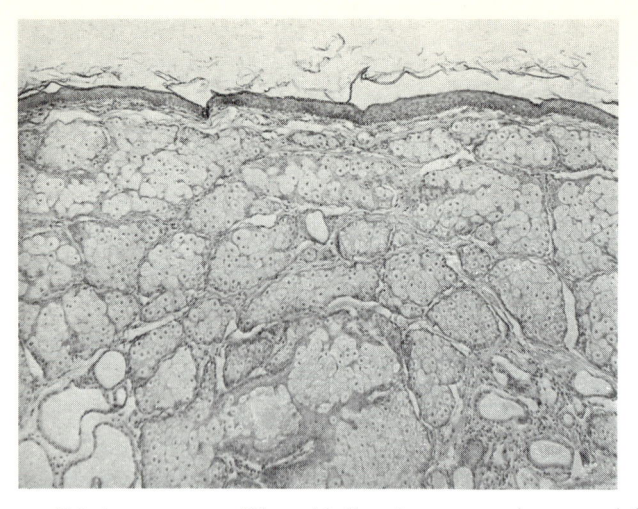

Fig. 15.—Skin in a teratoma. The epithelium is squamous in type and there is well-marked keratinization. Closely packed sebaceous and sweat-glands are present in the 'dermis'. (× 80.)

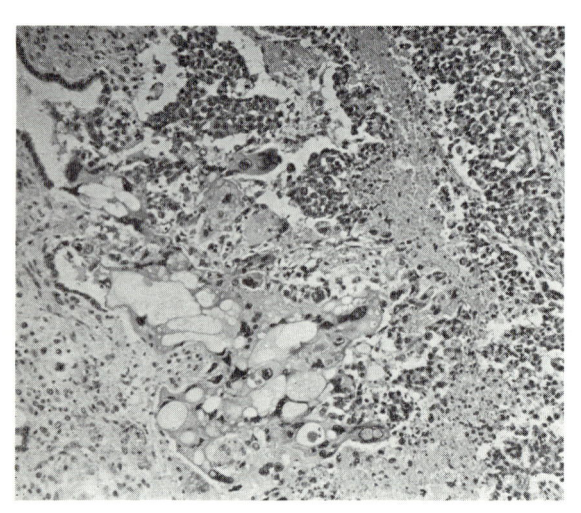

Fig. 16.—Choriocarcinoma of the testis. In this tumour there are sheets of cells closely resembling syncytiotrophoblast. This type of tumour often produces gonadotrophic hormone. (× 80.)

phenomenon than progression, but, because of its unusual nature, it has attracted much more attention in the scientific literature. It is an undoubted fact that there have been cases in which tumours judged to be malignant by all the available criteria have ceased to grow and have disappeared. In some cases, notably examples of neuroblastoma, a malignant tumour of primitive nerve-cells seen most often in the adrenal medulla of children, comparison of serial biopsies has shown a change from the closely packed, ovoid, ill-differentiated cells of neuroblastoma to the large cells showing close histological resemblance to normal nerve-cells of the benign counterpart, ganglioneuroma. Similar changes have also been observed in the so-called embryonic tumours of the liver and kidney in children, hepatoblastoma and nephroblastoma. It is difficult to conceive of evolutionary changes in the cells of the tumour of the type discussed above in connexion with progression having such an effect. In progression it is reasonably postulated that the better adapted, more rapidly growing cells come to dominate the population; the well-differentiated cells of a ganglioneuroma are less rapidly growing than those of a neuroblastoma and would be unlikely to replace them. A more probable explanation is that the cells of these tumours are still to some extent susceptible to the mechanisms which control differentiation and that at some stage in the life cycle of the tumour, or of the child, the control mechanisms become sufficiently powerful to induce fuller differentiation and slower growth in the tumour cells.

A second mechanism which may be invoked to explain regression is that of immunity (CHAPTER XIII). Cases have been described in which overt secondary deposits have decreased in size following the removal of a primary tumour, and it has been suggested that in such instances the immune mechanisms were overwhelmed by the large number of cells in the primary lesion, but once this was removed, were able to destroy the secondary deposits. In other cases, particularly in choriocarcinoma of the testis, widespread secondary deposits of a lesion histologically identifiable with some certainty as of testicular origin have been found, but after careful search the only lesion in the testis has consisted of scar tissue. Here the suggestion is that the immune processes have been able to destroy the primary tumour but not the secondary deposits. It is probable that the development of a tumour depends in some measure on the absence of an effective immune response. It follows from this hypothesis that recovery of immune potential or perhaps enhancement of immune potential may lead to the destruction and elimination of established tumour cells in rare instances. Regression is well established in the case of Burkitt's lymphoma in which there is a complex of aetiological factors including both an external virus and the immune system of the host (CHAPTER XI).

Unfortunately at present regression of tumours can only be observed, it cannot be predicted. It is far too uncommon to be expected and we can do nothing to bring it about. One hopes that in the future it may be possible to devise means of encouraging this most desirable phenomenon.

CHAPTER VIII
ONCOGENESIS

AN understanding of the origin of tumours, oncogenesis, requires a study both of the aetiological factors concerned in tumour development and also of the changes in the cells of the body which result in a conversion from a normal functioning somatic cell with a capacity for growth only within strictly defined limits. The preceding chapters have dealt with some of the changes in cell function which are characteristic of the neoplastic state, and the succeeding chapters will comprise a consideration of the agents and factors which have been shown in clinical, epidemiological, and experimental studies to play a causative role in tumour formation.

Discussion of the causes of tumours differs significantly from discussion of the causes of some other diseases such as infection. In the case of infective disease the production of a clinically apparent disease state in the patient depends on the presence of an infecting organism, and on the reaction of the body to invasion by the organism. The two factors have been compared to the seed and the soil; the nature of a plant depends on the nature of the seed which is planted, but the size and development of the plant and even whether it grows at all depend on the nature of the soil in which it is planted. In the case, for example, of tuberculosis, many individuals acquire a few tubercle bacilli early in life, but in most cases the defence mechanisms of the body control the invasion without the development of clinical disease. Factors which impair bodily resistance, such as overcrowding, inadequate or faulty nutrition, metabolic disease, or other infections, affect the soil and hence affect the reaction of the body to infection. However, in the absence of tubercle bacilli, no matter what the general state of the body may be, the clinical infection tuberculosis cannot occur. In philosophical terms the presence of the specific micro-organisms is a *necessary* cause of tuberculosis although in the presence of a good defence mechanism the infection may not develop and the presence of the organisms alone is not a *sufficient* cause for the clinical disease. The accessory factors, while of causal significance, are neither necessary nor sufficient causes of tuberculosis.

In the case of neoplastic diseases the situation is inverted. No agent or factor has been found despite extensive searches which is a *necessary* cause of neoplastic disease. This is a fact of the utmost importance; the absence of a necessary cause implies that it is illogical to speak of '*the* cause of cancer', and it is illogical and incorrect to search for 'the cure of cancer', rather we must try to understand the complex of aetiological factors and to apply our knowledge in a search for preventive and curative measures. Also in contrast to the position in infectious disease, there appear to be factors which can be *sufficient* causes of neoplastic disease. Irradiation, in sufficient dose, will cause the development of neoplastic disease in most individual animals exposed to it. Similarly, painting the skin with tar will result in the production of tumorous overgrowth of the skin epithelium and eventually in the formation of skin cancers. Mostly, however, the development of neoplastic change in the cells of an individual depends on the interaction of a number of factors both external and internal. Some cigarette smokers develop lung cancer, but not all; some persons exposed to large doses of ionizing irradiation develop tumours, but not all. The reasons for the difference in response to oncogenic agents are manifold. The genetic constitution of the individual plays a part; stomach cancer is relatively common and breast cancer rare in the people of Japan, and in the Japanese people living in California and Hawaii compared to the experience of people in Europe and North America. Probably the state of the immune mechanism is important; second malignant tumours are more common in individuals who have neoplastic disease of the reticulo-endothelial system, and tumours are commoner in those who are treated for long periods with immunosuppressive drugs. We are confined in our clinical practice by our lack of detailed knowledge of these complex interactions and can often only apply relatively crude measures of prevention.

The means by which the change from a normal cell to a neoplastic cell capable of multiplication and spread is effected are also complex. Experimental studies have shown that some carcinogenic chemicals fall into one of two classes, initiating agents and promoting agents. If an initiating agent is applied to the skin of a rabbit no discernible effect is produced, there is no proliferation of skin epithelium, and no cytological changes in the cells can be seen. Similarly if a promoting agent is applied there are no overt changes and in neither case does neoplastic growth arise. If, however, the application of an initiating agent is followed by the application of a promoting agent, but not vice versa, a crop of papillomata and later of carcinomata will develop. These observations have led to the elaboration of a two-stage mechanism of carcinogenesis in which it is postulated that different aetiological agents may be responsible for the two separate stages in the development of malignant neoplasms. Most agents which have been used in experimental carcinogenesis have the capacity to act either as an initiator or as a promoter, although the degree of activity in each respect may differ. This theory helps to explain the difficulty of determining causal agents in naturally occurring tumours. If factors A and B are initiating and factors C and D are promoting agents, tumours will develop in the combinations A followed by C, A followed by D, B followed by C, and C followed by D, but individuals exposed to A or B or C or D alone will not show tumour formation. If these factors are, as is likely in life, not double but multiple, the epidemiological problem of sorting them out, unless the effect is very striking as in the case of cigarette smoking, becomes almost impossible.

A further complication has arisen following epidemiological studies over the past 20 years. If the incidence rate of a tumour is analysed relative to age it is found that, for the majority of neoplasms occurring in adults, the relationship between the two follows a power law:

$$I = kt^r,$$

where I is the incidence, k is a constant depending on the number of cells at risk in the organ concerned and on the effect of environmental carcinogenic factors, and t is the age in years. The exponent, r, lies between 4 and 7. It can be shown by mathematical analysis that this relationship will occur if the development of tumours is dependent on a number of changes, $r+1$, in the cells of the tissues concerned. The number of changes is generally between 5 and 8 although a modification of the theory allows a reduction to between 3 and 6 changes. Support is given to this concept by the few instances in which several different changes can be identified in the body. The best example of this is in the case of colonic cancer. It is commonplace to observe polyps in the colon; these are infoldings of the colonic mucosa with a vascular connective-tissue core covered by cells which are identical in appearance to the cells of the normal colon. This can be designated stage I. Stage II consists of a polyp similar to that of stage I except that in some areas the cells are less well differentiated, instead of being mucus-secreting cells containing vacuoles with basal nuclei the cytoplasm is eosinophilic and the nucleus more central in position. The abnormal cells are, however, confined to the mucosa and the lesion is termed 'adenoma malignum' (*Fig.* 8). Stage III shows the development of neoplastic potential in the epithelial cells which show multiplication and extension into the stroma of the polyp. Two stages of the oncogenic process can be seen in many situations in the body as carcinoma-in-situ and overt carcinoma (CHAPTER VI). Further evidence in support of this multistage hypothesis has been given by the observation that the relationship between age and incidence of latent carcinoma of the prostate, presumed to be an earlier stage in oncogenesis, follows a power law with an exponent much smaller than that for overt clinical prostatic cancer. In the case of polyposis coli the individual carries a gene responsible for the development of numerous polyps throughout the colon. This may be regarded as a gene which has the same effect as several of the earlier stages in carcinogenesis in this organ, and if the age incidence of colonic cancer in individuals carrying this gene is studied it is again found that the exponent in the power relationship is less than that for clinical colonic cancer.

In experimental studies the number of animals studied and the duration of the experiments do not usually lend themselves to analyses of this sort. It has, however, been shown recently that a power relationship of similar type can be observed when animals are exposed to carcinogenic agents for prolonged periods.

These two theories, the two-stage hypothesis and the multistage hypothesis, are derived by different methods, the one on the basis of the experimental production of tumours, and the other on epidemiological studies. The two are, however, not mutually exclusive. We do not know what changes may take place in a cell during the process of initiation or what further changes may occur during promotion, and it is reasonable to suggest that in each instance a number of changes caused by the same external or internal agent may be necessary. If this is so the sum of x changes in initiation and y changes in promotion gives a total of $(x+y)$ which may well equal $(r+1)$, the total reached by analysis of epidemiological data.

The role of immune deficiency in oncogenesis is still uncertain. While it is certain that tumours arise from cells which have undergone changes in the genetic material, it is also possible that a change in the immunological mechanism may be necessary. This could be represented in the mathematical analysis by one of the sequential factors which give rise to the power law.

In this central problem of general tumour pathology any discussion must be in the nature of an interim report. We can accept with some assurance that the essential changes of carcinogenesis occur within single cells and it has been shown by genetic analysis that many tumours do indeed derive from single parent cells. Many agents are known to have the capacity of inducing tumour formation and there are many factors which operate in defence of the body against the transformation of cells from the normal to the neoplastic state. It is also probable that a sequence of changes is necessary, probably in the genetic material of the future tumour cell because the tumour acts as a population of neoplastic cells each of which inherits its capacity from a parent cell. Finally, we must remember that there is no 'cause' for cancer in the sense of a necessary cause which if it were eliminated would eliminate this disease, or indeed which if eliminated would eliminate one type of cancer. Lung cancer is seen in non-smokers, leukaemia is seen in those who have never been exposed to radiation.

CHAPTER IX
GENETICS AND TUMOURS

OUR concept of genetics as a branch of human knowledge and our use of this knowledge in trying to reach an understanding of the mechanisms of human disease have undergone drastic and far-reaching changes in the past 20 years or so. The molecular biologists have taught us to think in terms of the basic genetic material, the DNA of the cell nucleus, in which genetic information is encoded by the arrangement of the bases thymidine, cytosine, guanine, and adenine. The parts of the genetic material which are active in a cell at any particular time depend on the action of repressing substances and of special operator genes whose role is to control the activity of further stretches of genetic material (CHAPTER V). Some of this control is relatively permanent and is probably mediated by proteins such as histone which form part of the chromosomal material, other parts of the controlling mechanism are responsive to fine changes in the chemical constitution of the cell cytoplasms and of the surrounding tissue fluids. Effect is given to the genetic information first by transcription to RNA, a similar linear macromolecule to DNA, which passes from the nucleus to the cytoplasm and there, with the ribosomes and special molecules of transfer RNA, acts as a template upon which the sequence of amino-acids which makes up a protein molecule is built.

In a study of tumour pathology we are concerned with the way in which the genetic constitution of the individual cell, the genotype, interacts with the environment both within and without the body, in such a way as to develop into a neoplastic entity. Consideration of viruses and tumours, for example, must include discussion of the ways in which the genetic material of the virus interacts with that of the host cell to induce neoplasia. It is no longer sufficient to say merely that the virus makes the cell neoplastic. A further genetic concept which must be introduced to our ideas on tumour development is that a malignant neoplasm, which is free from the controlling constraints of the host, can be regarded as a separate parasitic population of cells which is a dynamic entity capable in turn of responding by adaptation to the stresses put upon it by the environment. The development of resistance to chemotherapeutic agents and the phenomena of progression and regression can in some instances be understood most easily as a manifestation of evolutionary adaptation.

THE GENERAL PATHOLOGY OF TUMOURS

Many of the aspects of general tumour pathology which are to be discussed in other chapters of this book have genetic implications or are derived from genetic concepts. In the field of experimental pathology great benefit has been gained by the development, by selective breeding, of strains of laboratory animals which are particularly prone to develop tumours of some particular type, or which are responsive to some particular oncogenic agent. The differences in susceptibility of different species of animals to tumours of various organs and to particular types of tumour, such as the Sertoli cell adenoma of the testis which is common in dogs or the melanoma often seen in grey horses, have their origin both in the genetic constitution of the species concerned and in the environment. The suggestion that the cellular system of immunity which is enjoyed by higher animals is an adaptation to the capacity for tumour development in vertebrates is a genetic-evolutionary concept which will be discussed in CHAPTER XIII when the relationship of immune processes to neoplastic disease is considered. In the remainder of this chapter I shall consider the relationships between genetics and tumours in terms of the concepts of classic genetics, genes, polygenic effects, polymorphism, and chromosomes.

SINGLE GENES AND TUMOURS

The origins of genetics lie in the study of the effect of single genes, short lengths of chromosomal DNA which are transcribed as units, and which, according to present-day theory, each lead to the production of a single protein or polypeptide molecule which may act as an intracellular control, as a structural element of the body, or as an enzyme. We have been accustomed since the work of Garrod at the beginning of the century to think in terms of 'one gene, one enzyme', and to try to relate the effects of genetic abnormalities and their effects in this way.

The list of neoplastic diseases which are associated with classic single-gene genetics is a short one (*Table II*). This list, although short, requires qualification. The citations of bilateral acoustic neuroma, carcinoma of colon without polyposis, phaeochromocytoma, multiple myeloma, and Wilms's tumour, nephroblastoma, imply only that some families have been described in which these tumours have occurred with a frequency and pattern which are indicative of the operation of a single-gene genetic factor. In most instances of these tumours no simple genetic background can be established and the risk of other members of the family developing the lesion appears to be small. The inheritance in the recessive mode of the closely related Letterer-Siwe disease and familial histiocytic reticulocytosis is also based on a few families and in most instances the cases which are seen appear to be sporadic. These two tumours are lesions of the reticulo-endothelial system and their mode of origin is probably more closely bound to the aberrations of immune development than is that of many other tumours.

GENETICS AND TUMOURS

A striking feature of this list of tumours apparently controlled by single genes is that the majority are inherited in the dominant mode, that is to say, a single abnormal gene in the pair carried on the homologous chromosomes is sufficient for the abnormality to become clinically manifest. This is in sharp contrast to the majority of genetically determined diseases in man in which a single abnormal gene, after transcription, can lead to the production of an abnormal protein, usually

Table II.—NEOPLASTIC CONDITIONS MEDIATED BY SINGLE GENES

Dominant	Basal-cell naevus
	Bilateral acoustic neuroma
	Blue-rubber bleb naevus
	Carcinoma of colon sine polyposis
	Cylindromatosis
	Diaphysial aclasis
	Multiple endocrine adenomatosis
	Epithelioma adenoides cysticum
	Keratosis palmaris et plantaris with oesophageal carcinoma
	Multiple lipomatosis
	Neurofibromatosis
	Phaeochromocytoma
	Phaeochromocytoma with thyroid carcinoma
	Polyposis coli
	Polyposis intestinalis—Gardner
	Polyposis intestinalis—Peutz-Jegher
	Retinoblastoma
	Self-healing squamous epithelioma
	Tuberose sclerosis
	Von Hippel-Lindau syndrome
Recessive	Familial histiocytic reticulocytosis
	Letterer-Siwe disease
	Multiple myeloma
	Wilms's tumour
	Xeroderma pigmentosa (or sex-linked recessive)

a defective enzyme, but the remaining normal gene on the other chromosome of a heterozygote can produce sufficient normal enzyme for the physiology of the body to remain unimpaired. It follows from this that the abnormal protein which is produced by transcription from the abnormal dominant gene leading to a tumour of this type is one which is physiologically active in some way, either by a direct action on cells in some situation or by interference with a normal repressing mechanism. In the majority of the genetically determined tumours there are lesions of one type of cell in many parts of the body: the bones in diaphysial aclasis, the nerve-sheaths in neurofibromatosis, the epithelium of the skin, its appendages, and the associated pigment cells in basal-cell naevus, cylindromatosis and epithelioma adenoides cysticum, and the blood-vessels in blue-rubber bleb naevus, and the von Hippel-Lindau syndrome. The syndrome of multiple endocrine adenomatosis and the association of phaeochromocytoma with thyroid carcinoma may similarly reflect an interference with the balanced interrelationships between the several endocrine glands (*see also* CHAPTER XII).

Tuberose sclerosis, epiloia, is a most interesting condition in which gliotic lesions of the brain, which may induce epilepsy and mental deficiency, sebaceous adenomata of the skin of the face, fibromata of the gums, angiomyolipomata of the kidney, rhabdomyomata of the heart, and cystic disease of the lungs associated with smooth-muscle proliferation between the air-sacs may occur. Any or all of these anomalies of the supporting tissues may be present in any combination; the mechanism by which this control of connective-tissue development occurs is unknown.

The three syndromes of colonic and intestinal polyps may represent the effects of three, or possibly four, genes at different loci, or the effect of abnormal genes different in different ways from the normal. In classic polyposis the lesions are confined to the large intestine and there is a very high frequency of malignant change. In the Peutz-Jegher syndrome the polyps are located in the small intestine and their histological appearance has been interpreted as that of malformation rather than adenoma and there is associated pigmentation of the skin; neoplastic change in the intestinal lesions is exceedingly rare. In the third type of polyposis, Gardner's syndrome, which is genetically distinct, the polyps are mostly in the colon and show a high frequency of malignant change, and there are associated epidermoid cysts of the skin and fibromata and osteomata of the jaw bones and in operation scars.

The only genetically controlled neoplasm which is consistently a malignant tumour *ab initio* is retinoblastoma, a tumour of the primitive retinal nerve-cells which histologically resembles the neuroblastoma of the adrenal medulla and medulloblastoma of the brain. The other lesions in this group are initially widespread benign lesions some of which may, over the course of years, undergo malignant change. It is probable that this is because the development of a malignant potential requires a number of changes in the genome of the cells as a consequence of external or internal factors, and that in these benign lesions which have a high frequency of malignant transformation some of these changes have been effected by the mutation which has given rise to the abnormal gene, and, especially in the case of polyposis coli, there is a vastly greater number of cells upon which carcinogenic agents may act. The 'premalignant' component of a gene may be present or absent. Tylosis, keratosis palmaris et plantaris, is a genetic anomaly inherited in a dominant fashion in which the affected individuals have greatly increased keratin deposition on the palms of the hands and the soles of the feet. In the vast majority of families affected by this disorder the inconvenience of physically repellent hands and feet is all that they have to suffer. In a very small number of families, however, the carriers of the tylosis gene, if they survive sufficiently long, develop carcinoma of the oesophagus and usually die from this cause in middle age. The mechanism of this gene action is unknown, and the difference between the more usual form of tylosis and this lethal aberration is quite obscure.

The single well-established genetic disorder associated with neoplasms and inherited as a recessive condition is xeroderma pigmentosa. In this condition the skin is normal at birth. After exposure to sunlight there is first drying and hyperkeratosis with erythema, and the development of pigmented freckles; later the skin becomes atrophic and the pigmentation becomes more diffuse, and finally squamous-celled carcinomata develop in exposed areas. The changes in the skin are related to an abnormal sensitivity to ultra-violet light, and it has very recently been shown that these individuals are deficient in an enzyme which is concerned in the repair of DNA molecules which have been damaged by this form of radiation. Presumably a sufficient exposure to this form of light can eventually lead to changes in the genome of the epithelial cells which have a neoplastic effect. It is interesting that in this solitary recessive preneoplastic state it can be shown that, in common with other recessive disorders, a deficiency of enzyme action exists.

Before leaving the consideration of single-gene genetics and neoplastic disease I would like to suggest that there may be other genes, as yet undiscovered, which may affect the susceptibility of individuals to disease without being evident in a benign form, and which may only increase the risk of tumour development. In the case of polyposis coli it is fairly certain that in time all carriers of the gene will develop colonic cancer. If, however, a gene has the effect of making the cells of the colon twice as susceptible to carcinogens in the intestinal contents, then many carriers of the gene will pass through a normal life span without developing colonic cancer. Detection and analysis of such a hypothetical gene present a problem of enormous difficulty but it is a possibility which must be borne in mind and it might account for some geographical variations in tumour incidence such as the high frequency of gastric cancer in the people of Japan.

POLYGENIC FACTORS

Many, probably most, of the characters which can be observed in man are the result of the interaction of a number of genes with the environment. The quantitative result of such an interaction is a distribution of values of the character which has the bell shape of the curve of the 'normal' distribution. Most values lie close to the mean and a frequency of excessively larger or excessively small values is very low. This is the type of distribution which is seen, for example, in height and intelligence. A similar form of variation probably exists in the character, susceptibility to tumour development, which at present we cannot measure, and it is likely that differences in cancer incidence in populations which live in similar environments may be related to differences in the gene pool and therefore to different average liability to tumour development. Such a mechanism would explain why not all cigarette smokers develop lung cancer, although they are exposed to similar carcinogenic environments, and also that in populations of experimental animals which are often highly inbred the response to carcinogenic agents is more uniform than it is in the human.

Members of a family group have similar genetic characteristics both in the expression of single genes and in the expression of the combined effects of groups of genes. It is possible that some of the 'cancer families' in which several individuals have developed tumours of some particular type are showing the effect of polygenic factors. It must be remembered, however, that very large numbers of families are observed, but that only the ones in which associations of this type are striking are reported in the literature. In England and Wales approximately 1 in 4 of the population die as the result of malignant disease. By random sampling we would expect that in 256 families of 4 individuals, in 1 case all would die of cancer, in 12 cases 3 would die of cancer, in 54 cases 2 would die of cancer, and in 108 cases 1 would die of cancer, and in 81 cases, over one-third of the families, none would die of cancer. The association of several cases in one family is therefore not unduly rare, and caution must be exercised in interpreting the occasional occurrence of multiple tumours in one set of brothers and sisters.

ASSOCIATION OF TUMOURS WITH OTHER GENES

One special example of this association, that of tylosis with oesophageal cancer in a small number of families, has been discussed already. A steady search for such associations has been made over the years with relatively little positive result. This is probably partly because such associations are rare and also because a study of very large numbers of cases is necessary if a small difference in susceptibility is to be detected.

Three well-established positive results so far recorded are the increased frequency of gastric cancer in individuals of blood group A, the increased frequency of tumours in patients with agammaglobulinaemia, and the increased frequency of the specialized Burkitt's lymphoma in children who have normal haemoglobin over those who carry one or two sickle-cell genes. In the case of the association with blood group A, the mechanism for the association is uncertain. It probably involves the release of blood-group polysaccharides from the cells of the gastric mucosa; either the polysaccharides of group-A individuals potentiate the action of ingested carcinogens or the polysaccharides of group-O individuals have some protective action. The relationship between agammaglobulinaemia and tumours is related to the reduced immunological capacity of individuals with this disorder and will be considered at more length in CHAPTER XIII. In the case of Burkitt's lymphoma, current thought on the aetiology of the condition suggests that a virus is concerned, and also that the presence of infection with the malaria parasite may be involved. The relative resistance of individuals carrying the genes for sickle-cell haemoglobin to the infection with this parasite may therefore, in an indirect way, help to protect them from the development of this disease.

The shortness of this section reflects our current lack of detailed knowledge of the mechanisms of gene action on the normal and abnormal functioning of the body. Inevitably the number of data available will increase, and a more detailed understanding will lead to a fuller comprehension.

CHROMOSOMES AND TUMOURS

It is well known that the genetic material of the cell nucleus is organized in a system of chromosomes, 46 in number in man, which can be seen in the mitotic cell at metaphase although in the intermitotic nucleus the chromosomal material is diffuse and active transcription of parts of it is taking place. The suggestion made at the beginning of the century that tumours were due to some simple aberration in chromosomes, a deletion or reduplication, has now been discounted by the majority of workers, and modern studies of the chromosome complement and form of malignant cells have been of little help in understanding the mechanisms of carcinogenesis. If the cells of a benign tumour can be cultivated *in vitro* it is usually found that the chromosome complement is that of normal cells. Cultivation of these cells is difficult and the majority of reported observations have been on cell cultures of malignant tumours. These frequently show a grossly abnormal karyotype with a chromosome number less than or, more often, much greater than that of normal cells. In a few tumours so-called 'marker chromosomes', atypical chromosomes of characteristic morphology, have been recorded, but in general the pattern varies from one tumour to another. In some cases serial biopsy and chromosome analysis have shown changes in the chromosome constitution of the neoplastic cells. These phenomena may be explained by reference to the concept that the tumour is a population of independent cells. To a great extent the functional capacity of human cells is not necessary to the tumour cell, nutrients are supplied by the host, and specialization of structure and function is not required. The cells of the malignant population can therefore adapt to changes in the environment either due to changes in the host or due to the proximity of other tumour cells by a wide variety of genetic adaptations which may include reduplication or loss of chromosomes. Furthermore, such cells never enter a meiotic cycle of cell division and therefore the need for pairing of chromosomes is lost and because of their independence of control, exercised *inter alia* by the immune mechanisms, a variety of forms can develop. A clinically apparent tumour 5 cm. in diameter contains about 6×10^{10} cells. This corresponds to about 30 or, more probably, because of cell loss and degeneration, 50 or 60 series of cell divisions which afford ample opportunity for evolutionary changes to occur. The chromosome constitution of tumour cells has been used on occasion to assess the malignancy of meningioma but this is, as yet, far from being a routine procedure.

There is one chromosome anomaly which is consistently associated with a particular type of malignant disease. This is the 'Philadelphia chromosome', which is a small fragment believed to represent a deletion of one arm of one of the small acrocentric chromosomes which is conventionally numbered 22. This aberration is consistently seen in chronic myeloid leukaemia and has also been observed in patients with polycythaemia who have subsequently developed the haematological and clinical features of myeloid leukaemia.

A number of clinical syndromes are associated with an abnormal chromosome constitution. In one of these, Down's syndrome, formerly designated 'mongolism', there is an increased likelihood of the development of acute leukaemia. The basic chromosome anomaly in these patients is that there is an extra small acrocentric body, probably an extra chromosome 21, and it is likely that the genes carried on this chromosome include some which are concerned with leucocyte growth multiplication and development. A somewhat increased frequency of gonadal tumours has been observed in patients with the chromosome anomaly of Turner's syndrome in which the karyotype includes only one X chromosome. It is, however, possible that in those patients the intra-abdominal situation of a gonad which is incompletely developed as an ovary is the most important factor.

CHAPTER X

ENVIRONMENTAL FACTORS IN TUMOUR FORMATION

THE development of neoplastic disease can in many instances be related to factors external to the individual, derived from the environment in which he lives. These environmental carcinogens have been subjected to intense investigation both in the laboratory and in the field of epidemiology in order to increase our knowledge of tumour development and also in attempts to reduce the incidence of tumours by eliminating and avoiding carcinogenic hazards. The agencies concerned fall into two groups, physical and chemical, and in many instances have been found to be associated with particular occupations. The full story of environmental carcinogenesis is by no means yet known. It is certain that there are more substances to be discovered and the mechanisms by which external agents cause changes in cells are all too obscure.

PHYSICAL AGENTS

Two classes of physical agents are implicated in tumour formation, physical injury and the effect of radiation. In the present state of knowledge the latter is by far the more important.

INJURY

The response to injury of any part of the body, whether the trauma is acute or chronic, involves cell multiplication to repair the damage produced. The increased mitotic activity in the regenerating cells renders them somewhat more liable to undergo mutational changes and to evince the effects of such changes as neoplasm. There is surprisingly little clinical evidence to relate injury to tumour development although claims are frequently made that this, that, or the other tumour has arisen in a site which has in the past been subjected to a blow, and in many cases a tumour mass is noticed when attention is drawn to the area by a minor injury. The argument falls down when patients with minor injuries are followed and the frequency of tumours in the injured parts is found not to differ significantly from that in the non-traumatized population. There are a few examples of neoplastic disease which are recognizably related to specific long-continued trauma. It was the habit of members of some groups in northern India to carry with them, under their clothes, a small brazier full of burning charcoal to offset the extreme cold of the winter. In some cases a squamous-cell carcinoma arose in the abdominal skin adjacent to the brazier as a result of the continued thermal stimulation of the local epidermis. A second type of long-continued irritation is seen in the skin adjacent to the ulcers of chronic osteomyelitis, and squamous-cell carcinoma of these areas is a well-known clinical entity. A similar mechanism can be invoked to explain the frequency of colonic cancer in patients suffering from ulcerative colitis. Parasitic infection of the bladder by the eggs of the worm *Schistosoma* is common in some parts of the world and the long-continued irritation of the bladder mucosa in such patients leads sometimes to tumour formation.

Other evidence of local injury as a cause or as a contributory factor in tumour formation is less satisfactory. It has been claimed that meningiomata arise more frequently at the site of head injuries, although this has been denied by other workers, and similar associations have been claimed in other situations. It is possible that the reaction to injury and the connective-tissue changes of the repair process may provide a nidus in which metastatic growth occurs more easily although this is more often seen in connexion with surgical incisions made for the treatment of tumours where tumour cells may be implanted at the time of operation.

An interesting physical factor which has been found to be associated with tumour growth is the implantation of plastic film. If a piece of plastic film is implanted in the connective tissues there is a risk of the adjacent connective-tissue cells becoming sarcomatous. This change is not seen if granules of plastic are implanted or if the plastic film has multiple perforations. It is suggested in this instance that the presence of the intact film interferes with the contact inhibition which cells exercise upon each other, probably by the release of chemicals, chalones, and that cell proliferation and overgrowth occur on the side of the film. If the film is perforated, the chalones can diffuse through and keep cell growth under normal control. Only one such tumour has so far been described in the human.

RADIATION

Cancer of the skin is more frequent in parts of the world where there is more and brighter sunlight, and protection to the individual is given by the pigment present in the skins of the indigenous peoples. The damaging radiation is in the ultra-violet part of the spectrum. Ultra-violet rays can penetrate the skin for a short distance and cause damage to the DNA in the nuclei of skin cells, thereby producing genetic changes in the cells. In the special case of xeroderma pigmentosa, a congenital skin condition in which tumour development following exposure to ultra-violet light is almost inevitable, it has recently been shown that

ENVIRONMENTAL FACTORS IN TUMOUR FORMATION

the enzymes necessary for repair of DNA are deficient and that damage once produced cannot be healed (CHAPTER IX).

The more penetrating and more powerfully ionizing radiation of shorter wavelength, X-rays and gamma-rays, and the ionizing alpha- and beta-particles given off by natural and artificial radioactive atoms are of great significance in carcinogenesis. Over 400 years ago it was noted that the workers in the mines of Joachimstal and Schneeberg were prone to die of a wasting disease associated with pulmonary symptoms. We now know that this was lung cancer and it has been shown that the air of these mines contains a radioactive gaseous element, radno, which was inhaled over long periods by these workers. In the 1920s and 1930s it had been noted that radiologists, radiographers, and physicists working with X-rays which were developed about the turn of the century have been liable to develop skin cancers and leukaemia, although the screening precautions with lead and barium and the development of narrow beams of X-rays have now largely eliminated this risk. Therapeutic radiation has also been responsible for tumour development; X-ray therapy of the enlarged thymus of children has been followed by malignant disease of the thyroid which lies within the irradiated field, leukaemia is more common in those who have received radiation therapy for ankylosing spondylitis and metropathia, and tumours have been reported in the fields of tissue irradiated during treatment of malignant tumours. The use of thorium in treatment and as an adjunct to radiological examination has also been followed in many cases by tumour development. Even the small doses given during diagnostic radiology may play a part in cancer formation; the frequency of leukaemia and of solid tumours is greater in the children of mothers who have had X-ray examination of the abdomen or the pelvis during pregnancy than in children whose mothers were not so examined.

An occupational hazard of the inter-war years occurred in the use of luminous paint which contains a small amount of radium; the girls who were employed in painting clock dials used to lick their brushes to make better points and so ingested some radium which, because of its chemical similarity to calcium, was concentrated in the bones. Later the effects of this radiation were shown as bone sarcomata.

More recently, since the discovery of atomic fission and the development of atomic and hydrogen bombs and the growth of the atomic energy industry, large amounts of man-made radiation and radioactive elements have been introduced into the environment. The death-rate from tumours in those who survived the atomic blasts at Hiroshima and Nagasaki has been greater than would have been expected, and the increase in radiation from the fall-out after tests of nuclear devices has increased the general risk of neoplastic disease in the population of the whole world. A particular hazard is contamination with radioactive strontium, ^{90}Sr, which behaves chemically like calcium and is concentrated in the bones. This isotope has a half-life of 28 years and can give rise to bone tumours and to leukaemic transformation of the bone-marrow.

The mode of action of radioactivity and of ionizing radiation in causing tumour formation is that of damage to the genetic material of cells. The effect of radiation is to produce ions and free radicals in the tissues by knocking electrons out of their shells around the atoms; the recombinations made possible by this means alter the genetic material and produce mutations. There is a continuous background of radiation, partly from the cosmic rays which reach the earth from the sun and from space, and partly from the naturally occurring radioactive elements in the environment; even within our bodies a small proportion of the potassium is in the form of a radioactive isotope. It is not yet settled whether the small amount of background radiation plays any part in carcinogenesis and it has been argued that there is a threshold below which doses of radiation have no significance in tumour formation. Experimental evidence on this question is equivocal partly because of the difficulty in devising and controlling an experiment which would establish a small effect from a low dose of radiation. I think it probable that there is no threshold and that even a single photon of gamma-rays has a statistically very small but nevertheless finite probability of contributing to tumour formation in the cell in which it is absorbed.

CHEMICAL AGENTS

The history of chemical carcinogenesis is also of respectable antiquity. Pott, the distinguished eighteenth-century surgeon who is eponymously remembered for a fracture, a disease, and a tumour, noted the high frequency of scrotal cancer in chimney sweeps in 1775. This tumour is attributed to the oils in the soot which, in the days before bathrooms, invested the body of the sweep throughout most of his working life. In the early years of this century it was shown that tar painted on the skins of rabbits induced tumour formation and by 1915 pure chemicals which were carcinogenic had been isolated. There is a very long list of chemical elements and compounds which have been found to have carcinogenic activity, but before coming to a consideration of some of them and the way in which they act, there are a few general points which merit consideration.

Carcinogenic substances fall into a number of groups according to their activity in this respect. Some compounds in the pure state are capable of producing all the changes necessary for the transformation of cells from the normal to the neoplastic state. Others have either an initiating action or a promoting action, or both. They can induce either early changes or late changes in the carcinogenic process (CHAPTER VIII), and yet others function as co-carcinogens and act synergistically with other compounds to induce tumour formation. This co-carcinogenic activity may involve oncogenic factors other than chemicals; hormones, viruses, physical agents, and the genetic composition of the individual co-operate with chemical factors and with each other in tumour formation.

In the case of carcinogenic substances which have a local action, it is the substance applied which is presumed to have the carcinogenic effect, but when the effect is seen at a distance, for example in bladder cancer after ingestion of a carcinogenic chemical, the active compound may be a metabolite of the substance originally ingested. This metabolic process may also determine the site of action of carcinogenic substances administered in a systemic manner. The concentration of enzymes of all types varies widely from place to place in the body, and spatial differences in the effective metabolism of compounds which are quite closely related chemically can occur.

Two other alternative chemical actions which may be contributory to carcinogenesis are immunosuppression and activation of dormant viruses. CHAPTER XIII comprises a discussion of the role of immunity in tumour development and it is shown there that a defective immune mechanism may allow tumours to develop from cells which have undergone mutational changes. If the immune system is suppressed by chemicals this defence mechanism will be impaired and tumours produced indirectly. The question of dormant viruses, viral material incorporated into the cell and reproducing synchronously with the cell nucleus and having no overt effect, is an open one. If such viruses are present they may be stimulated into activity, which may be carcinogenic, by compounds not generally regarded as having this capacity.

Finally, caution must be exercised in the interpretation of the results of animal experiments and in the transposition of such data to human pathology. In the experimental field it is necessary to use doses of carcinogenic substances which will produce a high yield of tumours within a limited experiment. This factor means that carcinogenic substances of low activity are less likely to be detected; a very large experiment would be needed to show, for example, that cigarette smoking, which increases the risk of lung cancer in men by a factor of about 25, was carcinogenic as only about 1 in 20 of heavy smokers develop this disease, and an experiment including many hundreds of animals would be necessary to demonstrate the effect. In the contrary sense the large doses of carcinogenic substances used in the experimental laboratory may overwhelm the detoxicating and metabolizing capacity of the animal, and allow carcinogenic activity to be manifest when the amounts of these substances ingested in natural circumstances might be metabolized and excreted. An understanding of the level of a carcinogenic hazard requires not only experimental observation but also epidemiological study of the exposure and risk in the natural environment of men, where the doses are likely to be lower and because of the genetic make-up of the human the metabolic and other reactions may be different.

Many thousands of substances have been shown to have carcinogenic activity or are suspected of such activity. They fall into a number of chemical classes; some of the more important of these will be discussed briefly.

POLYCYCLIC HYDROCARBONS

The first proved carcinogenic activity of defined chemical compounds was seen in substances of this group. Chemically they consist of a number of rings of carbon atoms which have several double bonds and to which are attached hydrogen atoms and short aliphatic side-chains. They are present in tars and oils which have been formed from vegetable material in geological times and are also formed by combustion of organic material in conditions of poor oxygen supply. Polycyclic hydrocarbons are the active substances which produce scrotal cancer in chimney sweeps, cancer of the abdominal skin in mule spinners, and a variety of tumours in workers with tar and oil of various types. Such hydrocarbons form a part of the atmospheric pollution engendered by the inefficient burning of fossil fuels and it has been suggested that they may be formed in food by preservation processes such as smoking, and that they are the active agents in cigarette smoke.

1:2-Benzanthracene

1:2, 5:6-Dibenzanthracene

Benzpyrene

Naphthylamine

Many of these compounds are of the same size and shape as the purine–pyrimidine base pairs of the double helix of DNA and it has been suggested that their action may depend on disruption of the normal base sequence in such molecules.

ENVIRONMENTAL FACTORS IN TUMOUR FORMATION

ALKYLATING AGENTS, NITROSAMINES, AND AZO-COMPOUNDS

This group comprises a series of reactive compounds which are capable of inducing chemical changes in the bases of DNA. The alkylating agents are also useful in medicine because in suitable doses they interfere with cell multiplication to such an extent that they cause the death of multiplying cells and are used in the therapy of tumours.

$$\begin{matrix} R \\ \diagdown \\ N{-}N{=}O \\ \diagup \\ R \end{matrix}$$

Nitrosamines

Cytosine may be converted to uracil and adenine to hypoxanthine by the deamination and methylation reactions induced by these compounds with an effect similar to that of mutation. Many compounds of this type are known; some, the azo-dyes and the naphthylamines, are excreted by the kidneys and have been important causes of occupational bladder cancer. Others are detoxicated in the liver and may produce liver tumours.

ASBESTOS

The fibres of blue asbestos, a naturally fibrous rock, are thin and sharply pointed, and, when inhaled or ingested, can penetrate deeply into the lung or the wall of the gut where they settle and induce fibrosis and neoplastic transformation, particularly of the cells of the pleura and peritoneum. The associations between asbestos and pleural neoplasms were first observed in Africa where the rock occurs naturally and where asbestos waste was used for road making. In this country the association is seen more particularly in workers with asbestos and in those whose homes are contaminated with asbestos dust.

ALCOHOL

A high intake of alcohol has been found to be associated with a high frequency of carcinoma of the oral cavity, the larynx, and the oesophagus. The mechanism of this relationship is uncertain. It is possible that alcoholic drinks contain carcinogenic substances which may act locally, or, alternatively, it has been suggested that the detoxication mechanisms of the liver are impaired in alcoholism and that carcinogens ingested are not adequately metabolized. If the latter hypothesis were true, however, one would expect the frequency of tumours distant from the upper alimentary tract to be increased.

SMOKING

Epidemiological studies on humans have shown with almost complete certainty that the smoking of cigarettes is liable to produce carcinoma of the lung. The aetiological mechanism is related to the presence of carcinogenic hydrocarbons in the tars produced as cigarette tobacco is burned and to the effect of these compounds on the mucosa of the bronchi. The lower frequency of lung cancer in those who smoke tobacco in pipes and as cigars may be due to the lower frequency of inhalation of smoke, to the retention of tars in the pipe-stem and in the unburnt tobacco of the pipe and cigar, to the different chemical composition of the tobacco prepared for use in these different ways, and possibly to different chemical reactions at the lower combustion temperatures of the tobacco when it is smoked by these means. There is also an association between smoking and cancer of the bladder; in this case the likely mechanism involves absorption and excretion of carcinogenic chemicals.

ELEMENTAL CARCINOGENS

Some chemical elements, when used either as pure substances or in the form of simple compounds, have been shown to have carcinogenic activity. Arsenic, beryllium, chromium, zinc, nickel, and iron have all been implicated although the mechanism of action is uncertain. In the case of nickel the occurrence of cancer of the lung and of the nasal sinuses was found in a group of workers using a refining process which involved the formation of nickel carbonyl and which also used sulphuric acid which was contaminated with arsenic, so that the relative roles of the two elements are in dispute. Experimental tests have shown that iron in the form of saccharated iron oxide was oncogenic when injected into animals; this compound is used in human medicine in the treatment of iron-deficiency anaemia, but so far no proof of a similar action in man has been described.

MISCELLANEOUS COMPOUNDS

A wide variety of other compounds have been shown by animal experiments to be carcinogenic or have been implicated by epidemiological studies of tumour formation. In most cases the mode of oncogenesis is quite unknown. The list includes food additives for flavouring, colouring, or sweetening, cosmetics, therapeutic substances including the alkylating agents and immunosuppressive drugs and isonicotinic acid hydrazide, urethane, lactones and aflatoxin, an antibiotic-like substance produced by the fungus *Aspergillus flavus* which is a common contaminant of food and which leads to the development of primary liver tumours.

The nature of the environmental factors concerned in carcinoma of the uterine cervix is as yet unknown. This tumour is seen more often in parous women and especially in women who begin sexual intercourse early and have more than one partner. It is, however, rare in Jewish women whose husbands are circumcised early in life. It has been suggested that there is a carcinogenic substance in the smegma which accumulates beneath the uncircumcised foreskin and this contention receives support from the observation that carcinoma of the penis is rare in those who have been circumcised in early life.

OCCUPATIONAL CANCER HAZARDS

Much of the epidemiological data connecting tumour development with chemical and physical carcinogenic agents has come from studies of occupations which carry a high cancer risk. The miners of Joachimstal and Schneeberg, the chimney sweeps observed by Pott, mule spinners, radiologists, luminous paint workers, and physicists have already been mentioned. Great help towards our understanding of neoplastic processes and of the environmental aetiological agents which contribute to their causation has already been given by careful study of the medical history of industrial and other workers and I am quite certain that further useful data await collection. I shall discuss briefly some of the occupational hazards in this field which are currently of importance.

RADIATION

Workers and administrators in the field of radiation are well aware of the carcinogenic risks attached to radioactive materials and sources of ionizing radiation, and careful checking of techniques and monitoring of workers is the rule. The field is still open for further observation particularly in respect of the linearity or otherwise of the dose-response curves and the presence of a threshold below which radiation is safe.

BLADDER CANCER

Excretion of carcinogenic substances or of their metabolites in the urine is an aetiological factor of importance in the development of bladder cancer. The wide variety of compounds used in industry leads to risks far beyond that of dye-stuffs manufacture which was the first to be recognized. Rubber workers, cable workers, and chemical laboratory staffs have all been shown to be exposed to potentially carcinogenic substances of this type, and careful consideration of new processes involving unusual chemicals in any industry is essential.

ASBESTOS

The role of the fibres of blue asbestos in the development of pleural endothelioma has been mentioned above. Asbestos is used in a wide variety of industrial processes and requires careful control. Fortunately white asbestos, the form which is used for such ubiquitous materials as brake linings, does not appear to have this property.

THE GENERAL PATHOLOGY OF TUMOURS

INHALED CARCINOGENS

Workers in the furniture-making industry and in boot and shoe manufacture operate in an atmosphere which includes very fine particles of organic dust from the wood and from the leather used as raw materials. These dust particles are trapped in the nose and in the lungs, and give rise to an increased frequency of nasal and lung cancer in these workers.

MINING

The principal occupational diseases of coal-miners are silicosis and chronic bronchitis related to the inhalation of mineral dust in the air of the mines. There is a high incidence of stomach cancer in these workers but no adequate mechanism of causation has yet been put forward. On the other hand, rather surprisingly, there is a lower frequency of lung cancer in miners than in the general population. This is not due to early death from other lung disease nor is it related to differences in smoking habits between miners and other men, and it has been suggested that the chronic lung irritation by mineral dust leads to a state of immunological enhancement in the lung of the miner which leads to a better protective mechanism and to more ready destruction of cells which may become malignant.

CHAPTER XI

VIRUSES AND TUMOURS

VIRUSES are the smallest known living organisms and require for their multiplication that they shall be inside a living cell, because they use the existing enzyme systems of the cell for reduplication of their genetic material, DNA or RNA, and for the formation of the protein coat which is found on the surface of the virus particle. The intimate contact of the viral genetic material with the metabolism of the host cell makes it natural to suppose that viral infection may be linked with tumour formation. The mode of virus attack on normal cells also suggests the possibility that infection of tumour cells by viruses may lead to the destruction of those cells and hence to the cure of the patient.

The relationship between a virus and the cell in which it multiplies is a particularly intimate biological co-partnership and there may be both species- and cell-type specificity. A virus may grow only in cells of one type or one species or may be innocuous in one animal and oncogenic in another.

VIRAL ONCOGENESIS IN ANIMALS

Studies of neoplastic disease in animals have shown that in suitable circumstances viral infection can lead to neoplastic disease. In the last decades of the nineteenth century it was observed that a tumour in dogs was transmitted from one individual to another, and there was some evidence that this transmission could be effected by cell-free filtrates. The tumour is the venereal sarcoma, a rapidly multiplying polypoid lesion which consists of small polygonal cells resembling reticulum cells, and is found on the penis of the dog and in the vagina of the bitch, and occasionally on the buccal mucosa. Recent observations have shown a constant abnormality of the chromosome constitution of the cells of this tumour, and it has been suggested that transmission is by the implantation of whole living cells. A separable virus has not yet been isolated.

Further naturally occurring tumours in animals in which viruses have been implicated are reticulo-endothelial lesions, lymphoma in cattle which can assume epidemic proportions in a herd, leukaemia in cats, and avian leucosis, a leukaemia-like disorder, found in flocks of domesticated birds.

By far the greatest contribution to the study of viruses in association with neoplastic disease has been made by studies on large numbers of laboratory animals mostly, for reasons of convenience, small rodents. In 1910 a fibrosarcoma of fowls was found to be transmissible from one individual to another by implantation and later by the use of cell-free filtrates. This is the Rous sarcoma, and the infective agent which has been preserved in laboratories all over the world has been designated the Rous sarcoma virus. Since then other viruses capable of causing leukaemia in fowls have been identified.

The next major step was the discovery of a virus which was responsible for the development of papillomata on the skin of the cotton-tail rabbit. This virus, the Shope papilloma virus, has been extensively studied and shows several interesting properties. In its natural host the lesions produced are multiple papillary tumours of the squamous epithelium which can be transmitted by contact from one animal to another but which rarely show malignant characters. If, however, the virus is used to infect domestic rabbits of an allied but different genetic constitution, the lesions are initially papillomata but progression to a malignant state and the eventual death of the host is common. On the other hand, if the virus is inoculated into the skin of animals of other species more distant from the natural host, infection does not occur and tumours do not develop. These observations indicate the specificity of the relationship between the virus and its host. In the natural host the virus parasitizes the skin epithelium but causes lesions which occasion only a minor degree of disability to the host; this is the optimal situation for the virus as the continual growth of the virus is assured and death of the host and hence loss of the viral population does not occur. In a host in which this relationship is less good, the effect of the virus is to cause a lethal condition which in natural circumstances is inimical to the survival of either member of the association. On the other hand, the virus is not capable of utilizing the metabolic processes of animals more distantly related to the natural host and tumours and viral multiplication do not occur.

The second significant laboratory observation has been that chemical carcinogenic agents and the Shope papilloma virus can be used in concert and will act synergistically. If the skin of a rabbit is lightly painted with tar in a dose which will not itself lead to the formation of malignant tumours and the animal is then given a small intravenous dose of virus, a profuse crop of lesions will appear in the tarred area and progression to malignant change is frequent.

One of the best known of experimental tumours has been mammary cancer in mice. Strains of mice have been developed in which almost all the females succumb during reproductive life to a malignant tumour of the mammary glands. In some strains this is a purely genetic phenomenon, but in others it has been noted that if the newborn mice are removed from the mother and suckled by a female of another strain, the expected tumours do not develop. Similarly it has been found that newborn mice of a non-cancer strain, if fed with milk from a cancer strain, develop mammary tumours in later life. The agent responsible for these phenomena is now thought to be a virus which is ingested in milk and which settles in the mammary glands. As the breast tissue develops during pregnancy and lactation, the virus multiplies and is excreted in the milk and produces neoplastic changes in the breast tissue, now stimulated to growth by hormonal action. In this instance the effect of the virus is apparently similar to that of an inherited character and it was thought for a long time that the phenomenon was genetic in nature.

Other types of 'vertical transmission' of virus which mimic hereditary processes have also been described. The virus may be transmitted in the ova or the sperm or may pass to the foetus across the placental barrier. Many of the naturally occurring oncogenic viruses pass from one animal to another in this fashion.

More recently other viruses capable of producing tumours in laboratory animals have been discovered. One of the most interesting and most scientifically productive of these has been the polyoma virus which can induce the development of a variety of connective-tissue lesions in mice, rats, and hamsters. These lesions may be potentiated by chemical carcinogens and also by the action of doses of radiation usually too small to be oncogenic alone. Further studies have shown that viruses which are natural parasites of higher mammals can, in the laboratory, produce tumours in experimental animals. A virus isolated from monkey cells, Simian Virus 40, and a variety of adenoviruses from human material have been found to have these properties.

Currently there is an extensive study of viral oncogenesis in primates in which many animals have been inoculated with a variety of viruses in infancy and are being kept under observation. This is a long-term study from which positive results cannot be expected for some years.

The laboratory study of the role of viruses in tumour development has proceeded at a much greater rate than has the application of such studies to human disease. The reasons for this difference are twofold. First, laboratory experiments are designed to give reasonable chance of success and viruses which show signs of an oncogenic capacity are studied extensively in species and strains which are convenient for laboratory use, and in which tumours appear prone to develop. This is a perfectly correct attitude, for the laboratory worker is primarily concerned with trying to understand the mechanisms of viral carcinogenesis and he sets up his experiments with specific questions in mind. Secondly, it is possible in laboratory work to design experiments which will enable Koch's postulates for the identification of an infective agent to be listed. It is possible to inoculate large numbers of animals with material from a tumour treated in a variety of ways. Such investigations in humans, where the risk to the recipient is that of developing a lethal malignant tumour, are not possible for obvious ethical reasons and the very rare reports of such investigations have been made in the expectation of negative results.

VIRAL ONCOGENESIS IN MAN

The only tumour of humans in which a simple viral aetiology is apparent is the common wart, verruca vulgaris. This is a benign lesion of the skin consisting of a papillary overgrowth of the squamous epithelial cells of the epidermis and is seen mainly on the hands of children and on the soles of the feet. The lesions are usually multiple and it is common to observe lesions on two patches of skin which are frequently in contact, such as the adjacent surfaces of two fingers. Malignant change in these lesions is exceedingly uncommon. The method by which the virus induces cell proliferation is not known. It is probable that the effect of the virus is one of irritation to which the epidermal cells respond by overactivity in the only mode of activity which they have, that of cell multiplication and keratinization. Such accentuation of the normal activities of cells is also seen in viral infections such as the common cold where the infected mucus-secreting cells of the nasal membranes overact with the consequent well-known streaming cold. Such overaction could well be due to an interference by the virus with the mechanisms of control of cell function.

A second human tumour in which a viral aetiology is very likely is the 'Burkitt lymphoma', although in this case the pathogenetic mechanisms are much more complex. The Burkitt lymphoma is a tumour of children which is common on the African continent and was studied and fully characterized only a few years ago. The lesions are found in the jaws and in solid viscera, such as the ovaries, as well as in lymphoid structures, and consist of sheets of lymphoreticular cells with a histologically characteristic 'starry-sky' appearance in the sections. It is unusual in that it shows a ready response to relatively small doses of such anti-tumour drugs as methotrexate. The geographical distribution of the lesion is dependent on climatic factors. It is seen in areas of up to 5000 feet altitude in Equatorial Africa, in areas of up to 3000 feet in subtropical Africa, and in areas up to 1000 feet in South Africa, and appears to occur only if the minimum temperature is greater than $15°$ C. and the minimum rainfall greater than 30 inches. Similar climatic conditions are seen in New Guinea and a similar tumour has been observed in that island. This distribution corresponds to that of a number of insect vectors of animal diseases and it was suggested that the development of this tumour might follow infection with some agent transmitted by insects. Extensive searches for infectious agents by examination of tumour tissue and by serological studies have shown an association between Burkitt's lymphoma and a virus which is also believed to be the causative agent in infectious mononucleosis, the E.B. virus. This disease is, however, common in temperate countries where the tumour is almost unknown and it is concluded that other factors are involved.

The current concept of the aetiology of this tumour is that it is the result of infection of the lymphoid tissue by the E.B. virus in an individual who is developing an immune reaction to the malaria parasite. The tumour is more common in children who are infected with malaria or who have been so infected and is less common in carriers of the sickle-cell gene who have a relative immunity to infection with that parasite. The fuller understanding of this relationship which may be as yet undetected in other tumours will undoubtedly help in a general understanding of tumours and tumour-like diseases.

In the case of other human tumours evidence of a viral aetiology or of a viral component in aetiology is less certain. The postulate of a viral factor in Burkitt's lymphoma led to extensive studies by direct electron microscopy and by cultural techniques in a number of tumours, and virus-like particles have been seen in the plasma of patients with leukaemia and with tumours of the reticulo-endothelial system, in sections of solid tumours of the liver and kidney, and in liposarcomata and osteosarcomata. Mycoplasmata, the 'pleuropneumonia-like' organisms which have some of the features of bacteria and some of those of viruses, have been isolated from the blood of a number of patients with leukaemia. As I have stated elsewhere, the few attempts to transplant tumours in men have been unsuccessful although in animal experiments the transmission of virus tumours is readily possible, and the observation of 'virus particles' and the culture of mycoplasmata are not positive proof of the aetiological nature of these organisms. A parallel may be drawn with the identification of *Haemophilus influenzae* as the causative organism of influenza before it was recognized that the true aetiological agent was a virus and that the bacteria represented an adventitial super-infection. In patients with malignant tumours there is some degree of depression of immunity and it is possible that the viruses seen and isolated may be adventitial passengers and not aetiological factors.

Serological studies have shown that there is evidence of infection with the herpes simplex virus in a greater proportion of patients with carcinoma of the cervix than in the general population. This, too, may be an example of a passenger virus infection or may be related to the known association of cervical carcinoma with a number of sexual partners, any one of whom may have transmitted the infection.

More suggestive evidence has come from epidemiological studies of leukaemia where it has been shown that cases of this disease tend to occur in clusters in time and space. When the date of diagnosis and the place of residence of large numbers of patients are analysed, it is found that a greater number of cases close together in time and space are found than would be expected on the basis of chance. These investigations are statistically difficult and are based of necessity on the date of onset of symptoms rather than on the date of initiation of the disease, but the tendency which has been shown in a number of studies suggests that viral or other infection may play some part in the aetiology of human tumours. The possible role of a viral component in a multistage mechanism of tumour development was discussed in CHAPTER VIII.

Recent studies in the field of tissue culture have shown that the cells of many organs in many animals are naturally parasitized by viruses which have no apparent clinical effect. Such viruses, passenger viruses, may be activated by external factors such as radiation or may simply become apparent when the less controlled cell multiplication of malignant disease comes into effect. A passenger virus can be contrasted with the 'driver' oncogenic virus which is seen in many animal tumours.

THE MECHANISM OF VIRAL ONCOGENESIS

A complete isolated virus consists of a genetic component which may comprise deoxyribosenucleic acid, DNA, which is the nuclear genetic material of the cells of higher animals and plants or ribosenucleic acid, RNA, which forms the messenger and transfer components of the genetic system of higher animals and plants. When a virus infects a cell one of two reactions occurs. The virus may act as a parasite and take over part of the metabolic mechanism of the cell which is invaded and use it for viral multiplication. When this process is complete the cell is broken down and fresh virus particles are released and are then free to invade other similar cells. The second type of reaction involves the incorporation of the viral genetic material into the genetic material, the genome of the cell nucleus. The viral DNA is then duplicated with the cell DNA at mitosis, virus particles are not seen in the cell cytoplasm, and cell destruction does not occur. It is more likely that in the development of tumours by the agency of viruses this second mechanism is operative and that the tumour produced depends for its properties on the change in character produced by the changed genome. This suggestion is supported by the observation of specific changes in the antigenic structure of cells transformed into malignant cells by viruses either *in vivo* or *in vitro*. The neoplastic cell produces proteins with antigenic properties which are independent of the origin of the host cell but dependent on the nature and the strain of the virus which is included in the genetic material of the host cell. Transition from the second to the first type of reaction can occur. In the case of herpes labialis the virus is carried for long periods in the cells of the buccal mucosa and only produces cell breakdown and the clinical lesion at intervals, often at times of reduced immunological capacity. The viral component of viral tumours is generally tightly bound to the tumour cell and is not released to form separate individual virus particles.

The concept of incorporation of viral genetic material into the genetic material of the host cell is difficult to accept in the case of the RNA viruses in which the genetic material is different to that of the cell in which the virus lives. This apparently contravenes the sequence DNA to RNA to protein which forms the usual mechanism of translation of genetic information to cellular expression. Very recently, however, it has been shown that enzymes exist which are capable of constructing a sequence of DNA bases on the template of a sequence of RNA bases, and it is therefore possible that a RNA virus may determine a permanent hereditable change in the genome of an infected cell.

Incorporation of viral genetic material into the genome of the host cell will result in a change in the character of the infected cell which may release it from the normal processes of control of cell multiplication and activity and hence lead to the assumption by the cell of properties which, in the environment of the body, lead to a malignant neoplasm.

An alternative possibility, as yet unproved, is that changes in the genetic material of a cell undergoing malignant transformation can result in a small segment acquiring the capacity to live a relatively separate existence. Such a segment would have the character of a virus which, in other cells, could have an oncogenic capacity. The complex system of inter-relationships between viruses and other cells makes it unlikely that evolution *de novo* has occurred but rather that these organisms have evolved from more complex cells.

VIRUSES IN TREATMENT OF TUMOURS

Clinical observations have been made on a number of occasions of the destruction of tumour cells by intercurrent virus infections. These have been transferred to the laboratory field where a number of viruses have been shown to have an onlytic effect on the cells of tumours developed in response to non-viral carcinogenic agents. In some cases this action has been shown to be potentiated by the use of immunosuppressive drugs which reduce the response of the host to the infecting viruses.

Three modes of use of viruses may be postulated. The organisms may invade the tumour cells in preference to the normal cells of the host and there multiply and cause the destruction of tumour cells. Secondly, the virus particles may invade the tumour cells and become incorporated into the cell genome and then produce changes in the antigenic constitution of the cells which may make them more easily destroyed by the natural immune defences of the host. Thirdly, viral infection, by stimulating the production of interferon or by enhancement of immunological potential, may act as a preventive measure against the action of other viruses which have oncogenic potential, or may increase the cell-mediated immunity action against the atypical tumour cells.

A few attempts have been made to induce viral infection in cutaneous tumours, usually by infecting melanomata of the skin with the virus of vaccinia, in some cases with the addition of measures intended to enhance the immune response. Occasionally this regimen has produced temporary regression of tumours, but permanent cure has not been achieved. The concept of using viruses as antitumour agents is a new one and so far clinical experiments have only been possible with viruses of low pathogenicity in patients with tumours which were beyond the reach of conventional methods of therapy. It is probable that in the future better methods of use of viruses will be found and in the more distant future again it is possible that the genetic constitution of viruses may be engineered so that preferential lysis of tumour cells is possible. This may sound fanciful, but already attempts have been made to replace deficient enzymes in individuals with genetic abnormalities.

CHAPTER XII
HORMONES AND TUMOURS

THE student of physiology knows that a great deal of the control of metabolism in the human body is effected by means of hormones, chemicals which are elaborated by the cells of the ductless, endocrine glands, and by 'endocrine cells' scattered in other situations, and are released into the blood-stream to be carried to other sites where they have their effects. A considerable degree of control of the activity of the endocrine organs is exercised by the pituitary gland, which produces trophic hormones which act upon the other endocrine tissues and which is, in turn, under the control of the brain through the hypothalamus. Variations in endocrine function are in general slow, and the system serves to maintain a state of homeostasis in which rapid variations can be produced by nervous activity. The connexion between this system and the problems of tumour pathology is complex and extensive; tumours may produce hormones, tumours may prevent hormone production, tumours may be induced by tumours and may rarely be dependent on them, and hormones may be used in the treatment of tumours.

HORMONES PRODUCED BY TUMOURS

The function of the cells of endocrine organs is to synthesize hormones. If the control of cell multiplication is lost, if a tumour is produced, and if the differentiation of the tumour cells is retained, an excess of hormone will be produced. The necessity for retention of differentiated activity (*vide* CHAPTER V) implies that the degree of multiplicative activity, of malignancy, will be relatively small and in clinical practice this is found to be the case. It is in tumours of the endocrine system that the boundary between hyperplasia and tumour is least well defined and, in general, the more malignant, more rapidly growing, and more widespread tumours of endocrine glands are not characterized by the production of excessive amounts of hormones. There are, of course, exceptions to this generalization; metastatic thyroid carcinoma can continue to produce thyroid hormone and the malignant chorionepithelioma produces large amounts of gonadotrophic hormone. In some instances aberrant hormone production may be associated with tumours of organs not usually regarded as endocrine in nature, and some of the general effects of tumours (CHAPTER III) are due to the effect of circulating chemicals produced by the tumours. The characters of hormonally active tumours of the several endocrine organs will be discussed briefly.

PITUITARY

The pituitary gland, the leader of the endocrine orchestra, has three main types of cell, acidophil, basophil, and chromophobe, in its anterior part, and cells of neural origin in its posterior part. The anterior pituitary produces hormones concerned with the control of growth and of the activity of the thyroid, parathyroids, adrenals, pancreatic islets, and the gonads and a hormone which is concerned with lactation following pregnancy. The posterior part produces the antidiuretic hormone which controls the flow of urine and oxytocic substances which act upon the uterine muscle. Overactivity of the endocrine function of the pituitary is, however, confined to two of the hormonal activities of this organ. An excess of growth hormone, which also has an effect upon the islet cells of the pancreas leading to reduced control of glucose metabolism, is seen in tumour and hyperplasia of the acidophil cells of the pituitary. If the patient is young and still growing the effect is to produce overgrowth, gigantism, while if growth of the body has ceased the effect is limited to the hands, feet, and face and is termed 'acromegaly'. This is an unusual disorder but is commoner than tumour of the basophil cells which is associated with the release of an excess of adrenocorticotrophic hormone and the clinical picture of Cushing's syndrome with oedema, hirsuties, hypertension, and electrolyte disturbances. Most often, however, this syndrome is due to tumours or hyperplasia of the cells of the target organ, the adrenal cortex, and not the pituitary itself.

THYROID

Most patients with disease due to an excess of thyroid hormone in the circulation are not suffering from thyroid tumours. In a few cases neoplastic disease of the thyroid is of the functional type, the cells can elaborate thyroid hormone, and the features of hyperthyroidism are seen. In such patients metastases retain the function of the primary tumour. This is useful to the physician and surgeon because in such patients the whole of the thyroid tissue may be extirpated without depriving the patient of thyroid hormone; the metastatic deposits concentrate radioactive iodine and can therefore be identified and treated with therapeutic doses of this isotope. In some cases the ability to produce a thyroid hormone which is functionally active may be lost but the capacity for concentrating iodine retained.

Recently a second thyroid hormone, calcitonin, which has the effect of lowering the level of calcium in the blood-stream, has been shown to be produced by the parafollicular cells of the thyroid. An excess of this hormone has been found in the blood of patients who have medullary carcinomata of the thyroid.

ADRENAL GLANDS

The adrenal gland, like the pituitary, is separable anatomically into two components, the cortex which is concerned with the production of hormones of the steroid type, and the medulla which is of neural origin and which produces catecholamines, hormones related to adrenaline.

Cortical tumours may produce an excess of steroid hormones which have effects on the metabolism of glucose, glucocorticoids, on the control of electrolyte balance, mineralocorticoids, and on the sex organs. In Cushing's syndrome, the commoner of the two endocrine

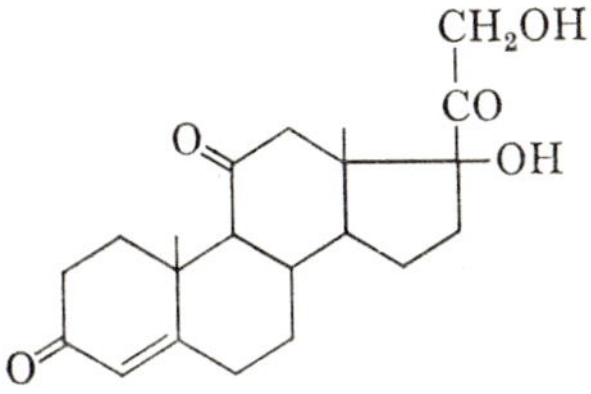

Cortisone

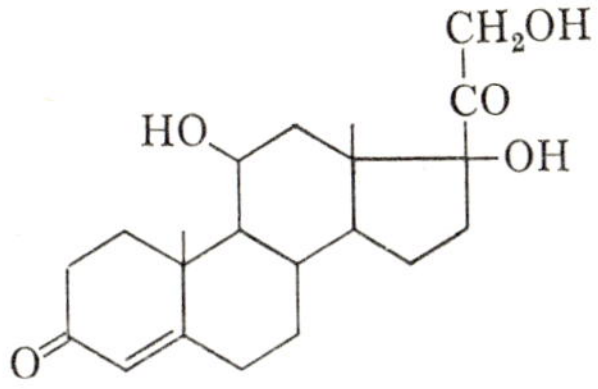

Cortisol

disorders associated with tumour or hyperplasia of the adrenal cortex, hormones of all three activities are usually present in excess. The clinical effects are obesity and oedema of the face, striae on the abdomen, resembling those seen in pregnancy, hirsutism in a male distribution, androgenic hirsutism, acne, and disturbance of mineral metabolism with hypokalaemia. Occasionally a single hormonal effect, such as masculinization, may be seen. The tumour may be benign or malignant in character and an indication of the degree of hormonal excess can readily be obtained by analysis of the urine for steroid hormones.

Less commonly, a tumour of the adrenal cortex secretes a single hormone, aldosterone, whose primary effect is on mineral metabolism.

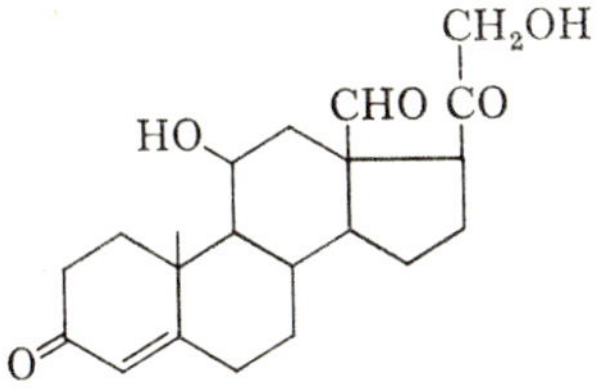

Aldosterone

The patient develops hypertension, muscular weakness, and polyuria, and is found to have a low level of serum potassium. Paraesthesia and tetany, related to the electrolyte disturbances, are seen in some cases.

Tumours of the adrenal medulla secrete large amounts of catecholamines which act on the musculature of small blood-vessels and produce hypertension which is typically, although not necessarily, paroxysmal in type. The majority of these tumours arise in the adrenal medulla,

$$HO\text{-}C_6H_3(OH)\text{-}CHOHCH_2NHCH_3 \qquad HO\text{-}C_6H_3(OH)\text{-}CHOHCH_2NH_2$$

Adrenaline Noradrenaline

but they can also occur in other collections of similar tissue such as the organs of Zuckerkandl which lie adjacent to the aorta in the abdominal wall and occasionally instances have been reported in the chest and in the wall of the urinary bladder. The more malignant tumour of the adrenal medulla, neuroblastoma, which is seen most often in children, is not usually associated with evidence of excess production of catecholamines although chemical analysis of such tumours has shown that these compounds or their precursors can be formed by the neoplastic cells.

PARATHYROIDS

In the case of the parathyroid glands only one hormonal activity is known. Tumours, usually benign in character, and hyperplasia of the glands are associated with an excess of parathormone in the blood-stream. The metabolic effect of this excess leads to release of calcium from a bound state in the bones and an elevation of the level of calcium in the serum and in the urine. Locally, in the bones, areas of bone resorption and of replacement of bone by fibrous tissue with many giant cells of the osteoclast type are seen. This manifestation is known as osteitis fibrosa cystica and may be associated with pathological fracture or with bone deformity. A similar lesion is also sometimes found in the mouth; an exuberant overgrowth of fibrous tissue in the gum and the jaw bones, the giant-cell epulis, has most of the histological features of osteitis fibrosa and in some cases there is elevation of the level of serum calcium. This lesion is, however, most often not associated with parathyroid tumour.

The excessive excretion of calcium in the urine may, in the presence of other predisposing factors, such as infection, lead to the formation of urinary calculi whch are occasionally the first clinical manifestations of parathyroid tumour.

THE PANCREATIC ISLETS

Approximately 10 per cent of the substance of the pancreas is taken up by a large number of islands of endocrine tissue which produce two hormones concerned with glucose metabolism, insulin and glucagon, and also hormones which influence the secretion of gastric juices. Tumours of the islets of Langerhans most often produce insulin and lead to a state of hypoglycaemia following periods of fasting. These tumours are usually benign. In theory islet-cell tumours should also be capable of secreting glucagon which acts antagonistically to insulin and in such lesions hyperglycaemia should be expected. Very few examples of such lesions have been recorded, but recently it has been reported that glucagon has been identified by immunofluorescent methods in the cells of islet-cell tumours associated with clinical diabetes.

The islet-cell hormone which has an effect on gastric secretion is the major aetiological factor in the Zollinger-Ellison syndrome of peptic and jejunal ulceration with hyperacidity associated with islet-cell tumour of the pancreas. A number of such cases have been reported and in several there have also been functioning adenomata of other endocrine glands.

THE GONADS

The ovary and testis are organs of dual function. They are the site of development of the germ cells—the ova and spermatozoa—which eventually fuse to form the new individual at conception, and, under the influence of the pituitary gland, they secrete hormones which influence sexual development. In the testis the interstitial cells secrete an androgenic hormone and interstitial-cell tumours have virilizing effects which are apparent if the tumour occurs before the age of puberty.

Oestradiol

Progesterone

Testosterone

Feminizing activity in testicular tumours is exceedingly rare, but has been recorded as gynaecomastia in cases of tumours of the gonadal stroma which resemble granulosa-cell and theca-cell tumours of the ovary. As might be expected, ovarian tumours are more likely to produce feminizing hormones of the oestrogen group and such compounds are produced in granulosa-cell tumour of the ovary and sometimes in thecoma. Masculinization is less common and is seen in the arrhenoblastoma which has tubular structures resembling the tubules of the testis and in hilus-cell tumour which resembles the interstitial-cell tumour. Masculinization may also be seen in association with tumours which appear to be of the granulosa-cell type.

The situation concerning the endocrine substances produced by the ovary and the testis is rather more complex than appears at first sight. The hormones are all steroids, all are based on the cyclopentanophenanthrene nucleus, and are closely related chemically so that one type may readily be converted into another. Furthermore, in the case of tumours the concentration of hormones in the blood is much higher than in a physiological state and the effect of very high doses of an oestrogen or of a progesterone may be paradoxically androgenic and vice versa.

THE CARCINOID SYNDROME

There are, scattered throughout the gut and in structures derived from the gut, cells which are present in the mucosa but which have the function of producing a simple hormonally active substance, 5-hydroxytryptamine, which, like some of the prostaglandins, has an effect on smooth muscle. Tumours of these cells are most often seen as the

5 Hydroxytryptamine

carcinoid tumour of the vermiform appendix. Small benign tumours of this type secrete hormone which passes in the portal system to the liver and is there rapidly degraded. If liver metastases occur or if the tumour arises in a situation without a portal venous drainage, the hormone reaches the circulation and produces a syndrome of diarrhoea, flushing, pulmonary valve stenosis, and bronchospasm. The commonest site of these tumours is the appendix; they are also seen in the small intestine and as one form of 'adenoma' of the bronchus, and they have been reported in teratomata of the ovary and as primary ovarian tumours.

PLACENTA

One of the functions of the placenta in its role of maintaining a suitable environment for the growth of the foetus is that of secreting a gonadotrophic hormone which controls ovarian and uterine activity. Tumours of the placenta, hydatidiform mole and chorionepithelioma, secrete large quantities of this hormone which is readily detectable in the urine of the patient and which provides a means of diagnosis and of control of treatment.

TERATOMA

The differentiated tissue of teratomata, as well as producing structures resembling those of the normal body, may have the functional capacity for producing hormones. The most important of these is the gonadotrophic hormone produced by chorionic tissue which is seen mainly in highly malignant teratomata of the testis. As has already been mentioned, carcinoid tumours with hormonal activity may also be found as a component of teratomata and oestrogenic activity has been recorded in a testicular teratoma.

PROSTAGLANDINS

The prostaglandins form a class of naturally occurring biological chemicals which appear to fall between hormones, enzymes, and vitamins in their physiological action. Chemically they are long-chain fatty acids with hydroxyl groups and double bonds towards the middle

Prostaglandins

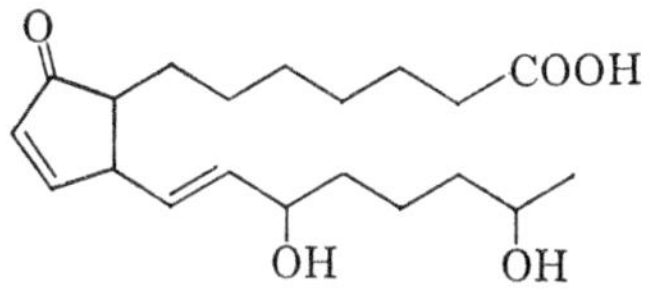

A_1

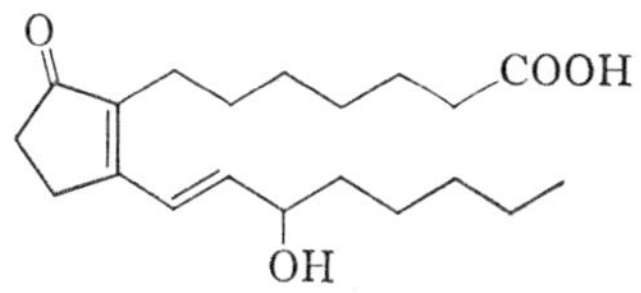

B_1

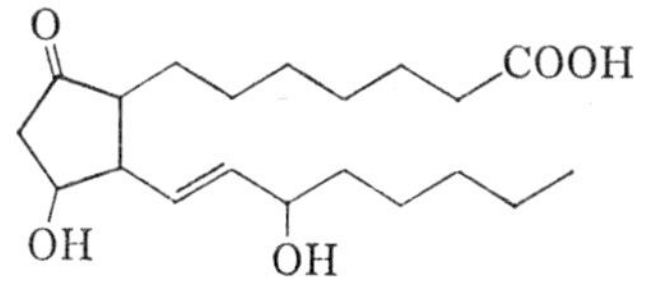

E_1

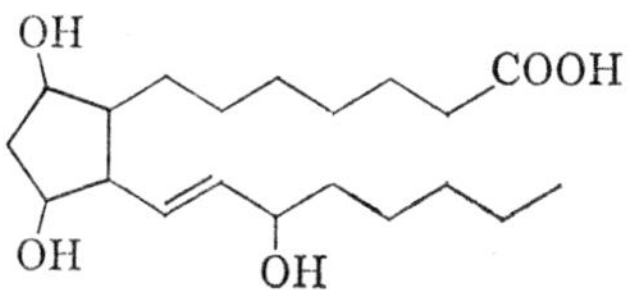

F_1

of the chain. Members of the group have been found in almost all tissues and their physiological effects are related to contraction and relaxation of smooth muscle, the maintenance of blood-pressure, the control of glucose and of fat metabolism, the metabolism of calcium, and the integrity of the blood-platelets. Research on this group of compounds is in active progress and many papers are being published each year. It has already been shown that a high level of prostaglandins is present in the serum of patients with medullary carcinoma of the thyroid, and high concentrations were found in the tissue of a series of aminopeptide-secreting tumours of the neural crest, foregut, and midgut. In some of these patients the high level of prostaglandin appeared to be associated with diarrhoea. It is probable that further relationships between these substances and neoplastic disease will be found in the near future.

PLURIGLANDULAR ADENOMATOSIS

In between 10 and 20 per cent of cases of the Zollinger-Ellison syndrome tumours are also present in one or more of the other endocrine organs, most often the pituitary and parathyroid, but also the adrenal cortex, and in some cases carcinoid tumours have been described. Tumours in several endocrine organs may be present at the time of initial presentation or they may, less often, develop sequentially. This association of adenomata in several endocrine organs shows a familial pattern and is thought to be due to the action of an autosomal dominant gene. It has been suggested that in some cases the tumour formation is apparent rather than real and that the condition is one of multiple endocrine hyperplasia perhaps under the influence of hormones from one tumour. A similar association, also possibly of genetic character, has been reported between phaeochromocytoma of the adrenal medulla and medullary carcinoma of the thyroid with, in some cases, multiple subcutaneous neuromata. This syndrome too is attributed to the effect of an autosomal dominant gene.

The existence of these syndromes of association of tumours of several organs underlines the incompleteness of our knowledge of the interrelationships between the controlling mechanisms of the various parts of the body, and also serves as a reminder that clinically and pathologically identical lesions may be the end-result of different aetiological processes.

ABERRANT HORMONE FORMATION BY TUMOURS

Hormonal activity, or apparent hormonal activity, may be exercised by a considerable number of tumours (*Table III*). In most instances the hormone concerned is a protein or polypeptide which would be synthesized on the template of a sequence of DNA bases which is included in the genome of every cell. It can be postulated in such cases

HORMONES AND TUMOURS

that unblocking of a segment of bases has occurred (*see* CHAPTER V), and that a new manifestation of differentiation becomes possible. The most frequently involved tumours are those of the lung. It has been estimated that about 10 per cent of patients with lung tumours show evidence of aberrant endocrine activity. Many of the other tumours

Table III.—ABERRANT HORMONE PRODUCTION BY TUMOURS

ACTH (adrenocorticotrophic hormone)	Oat-cell carcinoma of lung Carcinoma of: Pancreas, parotid, thymus, parathyroid, thyroid, prostate, ovary, colon, breast, testis Carcinoid tumours Phaeochromocytoma Sympatheticoblastoma	
ADH (antidiuretic hormone)	Oat-cell carcinoma of lung Carcinoma of prostate	
Hypoglycaemia	Fibrosarcoma Mesothelioma Rhabdomyosarcoma	Hepatoma Carcinoma of stomach Leiomyosarcoma
Hypercalcaemia	Hepatoma Carcinoma of lung Carcinoma of oesophagus	Lymphosarcoma Carcinoma of pancreas
Chorionic gonadotrophin	Teratoma Melanoma Carcinoma of lung Carcinoma of adrenal	Hepatoma Carcinoma of breast
TSH (thyrotrophic hormone)	Carcinoma of lung Tumours producing chorionic gonadotrophin	

are those of organs and cells which normally have an endocrine function, and it has been suggested that 'endocrine' cells are particularly prone to develop unblocking and are well equipped otherwise for the synthesis of hormonal proteins and polypeptides. The oat-cell carcinoma of the lung is regarded by some workers as a tumour of potentially endocrine tissue and would therefore fall into this group.

In many instances the responsible hormones have been identified in the blood-stream or in tumour tissue by pharmacological or immunofluorescent methods. In the case of hyperglycaemia the hormone postulated, insulin, is relatively easy to detect but some studies have failed to show evidence of insulin production. The tumours in question are usually large connective-tissue lesions and it has been suggested in such cases either that there is excessive consumption of glucose by the tumour or that substances produced by the tumour stimulate the pancreatic islets to produce an excess of insulin.

ENDOCRINE DEFICIENCY DUE TO TUMOURS

If an endocrine gland is destroyed by tumour the function of the gland will also be damaged and the clinical effects of endocrine lack may be seen. This is not a common occurrence. In most cases a tumour involving endocrine organs will be recognized and treated before endocrine deficiency is apparent and most endocrine organs are either large or multiple so that total destruction is unlikely. Chromophobe adenomata of the pituitary, which do not have endocrine activity themselves, may crush the normal organ and reduce the flow of trophic hormones but, more usually, the effects of pressure on surrounding structures become apparent earlier. Cases of diabetes due to destruction of all the pancreatic tissue by carcinoma have been described and there have been examples of Addison's disease due to destruction of both adrenal glands by tumour.

HORMONES AS AETIOLOGICAL FACTORS IN TUMOURS

In the experimental situation, if sufficiently large doses of hormones are administered for prolonged periods, or if hormone-producing glands are transplanted from their normal situations, tumours can be induced. Oestrogens can induce pituitary adenomata in some strains of mice and in some strains of rats; breast cancer can be induced in rats but less often in mice, and adrenal tumours are induced in rats but less often in mice. Large doses of oestrogen given to male mice also induce interstitial-cell tumours of the testis and in female rats and mice give rise to squamous-cell carcinoma of the cervix and vagina. The administration of other hormones does not produce many tumours, although progesterone can act as a co-carcinogen with some of the non-endocrine carcinogenic chemicals.

Castration is an easy procedure in laboratory animals and leads to a high frequency of tumours of the pituitary, adrenal, and breast, especially in the male, but protects the prostate against tumour development. Thyroidectomy also leads to a higher frequency of pituitary tumours. In the guinea-pig partial oophorectomy leads to a state of continuous oestrus in the operated animal and later to adenomatous polyps and carcinoma of the uterus.

In many ways the most interesting results have been obtained by splenic transplants. If a portion of an endocrine organ subject to pituitary control is implanted into the spleen and the remainder of the organ or organs is removed, the pituitary pours forth the trophic hormone which stimulates the transplant. Any hormones produced by the transplant pass directly in the portal circulation to the liver and are metabolized so that the negative feedback of hormone on the pituitary does not occur and under constant stimulation the transplant develops into a tumour. It is possible, although not yet demonstrated, that other causes of failure of negative feedback may operate in tumour development.

There are wide differences in response to hormone administration and surgical manipulation of the endocrine glands between species of laboratory animals and between strains within one species. These differences reflect the variation, due to genetic factors, in the response of cells to stimuli.

In the human, hormonal effects on the aetiology of tumours are less apparent. Oestrogen excess, whether due to the administration of these substances or to oestrogen-producing tumours, leads to hyperplasia of the endometrium which may go on to carcinoma. The long-term effects of pregnancy affect the tissue of the breast and the endometrium and tumours of these organs are more common in women who have not had children than in those who are fertile. The higher frequency of cervical cancer in parous women is more likely to be related to injury to the cervix and to sexual intercourse than to the effects of hormones.

HORMONE-DEPENDENT TUMOURS

A hormone-dependent tumour is by definition one which arises in an organ dependent on hormones and which requires hormones for its maintenance. Several varieties of breast cancer have been developed in laboratory animals which depend on circulating oestrogen and which regress if the supply of this hormone is cut off. The concept of hormone dependency is an attractive one because it offers a hope of treatment of tumours even when they extend beyond the reach of surgical excision. In the human, tumours of the breast are sometimes dependent on hormones in the circulating blood. In such cases remission can be obtained by treatment with high doses of oestrogens or of androgens, or by removal of the hormone-producing organs, the ovaries and the adrenals. Destruction of the pituitary gland by ablation or by the use of implants of radioactive material reduces the flow of trophic hormones and thence the hormonal activity of the other organs. In prostatic cancer a remission in the course of the disease may sometimes be effected by removal of the testes, but in the case of this tumour treatment with oestrogens, especially stilboestrol, is more effective. The use of hormones and of the ablation of endocrine organs in the management of malignant disease will be discussed in the last section of this chapter.

The exuberant endometrial hyperplasia which is seen in patients with feminizing ovarian tumours and latterly in those who are taking oral contraceptives can mimic neoplasm very closely. It is a convention that the lesions which regress when the source of excess oestrogens is removed are termed 'hyperplasia' and those which do not regress are called 'carcinoma'. Perhaps we should refer to the hyperplastic lesions as totally hormone-dependent tumours.

Unfortunately, apart from the possible case of endometrial lesions, hormone dependence is not absolute, and in the majority of cases the tumour sooner or later begins to grow again in an autonomous fashion. This is an evidence of the evolutionary and adaptive capacity of the parasitic population of tumour cells which can undergo change and in which a cell line capable of growth without hormones can emerge.

HORMONES IN THE TREATMENT OF TUMOURS

Extensive use of corticosteroids is made in the treatment of patients suffering from neoplastic disease of various sites. These hormones are used in large doses and appear to have a pharmacological rather than a physiological effect, and their action on tumours is related to their effects on the metabolism of the body as a whole rather than to a direct effect on tumour cells. Remissions may be obtained in acute leukaemia after the exhibition of corticosteroids, and these compounds are often used in association with other drugs. In brain tumours much of the symptomatology is often due to the presence of oedema in the surrounding brain tissue and relief of symptoms and time sufficient to allow surgical and radiotherapeutic effect may be gained. A similar pharmacological benefit is sometimes realized after administration of anabolic steroids related to the androgens. These have again a general effect on metabolism and thence on the reaction of the host to the tumour. More recently claims have been made that the administration of physiological doses of oestrogen to women past the menopause leads to an overall reduction in tumour frequency.

A more specific application of hormone therapy to neoplastic disease is seen in the use of oestrogens to control prostatic cancer and of hormones and endocrine gland ablation in breast cancer. In many cases of cancer of the prostate the disease can be held in check by the continuous

Diethyl Stilboestrol

administration of stilboestrol. This effect is potentiated by orchidectomy, but, as so often in tumour therapy, once the effective agent is stopped the tumour grows again and is often then not responsive to the hormone.

About one-third of all carcinomata of the breast are responsive to hormone treatment. It has been found that if there is a high urinary excretion of aetiocholanolone relative to 17-hydroxycorticosteroids the patient is likely to respond to oophorectomy and to adrenalectomy and hypophysectomy. Most of the responsive tumours occur in premenopausal women and in postmenopausal women in whom there is evidence of oestrogen excess. Androgenic hormones are useful in women 2–5 years after the menopause and in patients who show a positive response to castration. The female sex hormones, oestrogens, are more useful in older, postmenopausal patients.

CHAPTER XIII
IMMUNITY AND TUMOURS

DEVELOPMENTS in the field of tissue transplantation have led to an upsurge of interest in the phenomena of immunity, and to a great increase in our knowledge of the mechanisms of defence against external agents which the body possesses. It is now recognized that there are two separate but interlinked methods by which this defence is effected. The first of these is the system of humoral antibodies; specific chemical substances, the immunoglobulins, are produced by cells of the plasma cell family in response to antigenic stimulation. These specialized antibody-producing cells derive from parts of the lymphoid system which develop in the somatic tissues, and the antibodies are of particular importance in resisting infection by micro-organisms and in reducing the effects of toxins produced by these organisms. The second mode of immunological defence is that of cell-mediated immunity in which collections of sensitized lymphocytes and plasma cells are found around the foreign material. These cells take origin in lymphocytes which are formed in the thymus and migrate to the peripheral zones of the lymph-nodes. An immune reaction of the second type is characteristic of the host versus graft reaction in tissue transplantation, and both types of reaction are seen in the auto-immune diseases in which normal body cells are adversely affected by an aberrant immunological reaction. It has been suggested that part of the control of tissue homeostasis, the maintenance of normal numbers of cells in the various parts of the body, is one of the functions of the system of cell-mediated immunity. If this is the case, the important role of this system in carcinogenesis is apparent.

ANTIGENS

An immunological response of either type occurs following stimulation by antigens which are almost invariably complex protein molecules, each of which has a specific structure and probably a specific physico-chemical configuration. In some cases the antigenic state of the protein is modified by combination with complex polysaccharides. This is the case in the blood-group antigens which are of such great importance in blood transfusion. Every cell has on its surface proteins and protein groups which are capable of acting as antigens. In foetal life part of the process of development involves the creation of a system of tolerance between the immune system and the set of antigens which is formed on the cells of the individual. It is this tolerance, mediated by a specialized form of immune response, which prevents auto-immune reactions occurring in the normal individual. An immune response may be evoked by changes in the cells of the immune system (this is the case in most of the auto-immune diseases) by the introduction into the body of antigens foreign to the host and to which tolerance has not been established, or by changes in the antigenic structure of body cells. Foreign antigens are introduced in infection or in the surgical procedures of transplantation. The system of cellular antigens is unique to the individual and it is because of this system that grafts from one individual to another are rejected unless specific measures are taken to reduce the level of immunological response, either by irradiation or by the use of immuno-suppressive drugs.

The antigens of tumour cells may differ from those of the cells from which they arise in several ways. The cells of each tissue carry a variety of antigens among which are tissue-specific substances which can be used to identify the origin of the cell. In some tumours it has been shown that these organ-specific antigens are absent. If the theory that immune processes are concerned in homeostasis is correct, the absence of organ-specific antigens will impair the normal mechanism of control of cell growth and allow unrestrained growth, a characteristic of the tumour cell, to occur. Secondly, abnormal antigens may appear. These have in some cases been identified as antigens which are normally present in the foetal organ but which cannot be detected in normal adult tissues. One of these, an alpha-fetoglobulin, has been detected in the blood of patients suffering from primary liver cancer and may, rarely, be useful as a diagnostic test. Another, an embryonic gut antigen, has been found in the blood of patients with colonic cancer.

In the case of the tumours of experimental animals which are due to infection with specific viruses the antigenic structure of the tumour cell is altered in a way which is specific to the virus concerned. This antigen is determined by the genetic material of the virus which is incorporated into the genome of the host cell as well as by the action of virus particles living free in the host nucleoplasm and cytoplasm. In the case of non-viral tumours an irregular pattern of antigenic change is seen. The antigens of a series of tumours induced by a single carcinogenic chemical may differ widely, although when a single tumour is perpetuated by transplantation in syngeneic animals the antigenic structure remains constant.

IMMUNOLOGICAL REACTION TO TUMOURS

Tumour cells are subject to the immune response as are all other cells. In human subjects tumours could be transplanted from one individual to another in the few surgical experiments which have been thought to be ethically justifiable. Exceptions to this rule have been seen in the very rare natural transmission of tumour cells from a mother to her foetus in utero, in the case of tumours of trophoblastic tissue which are foetal tumours in the mother, and in the rare accident of a transplanted organ having in it an undetected developing neoplasm. Each of these exceptions has an immunological explanation. The foetus in utero is in an unusual immune state in that it is developing tolerance to its own tissue cells; the implanted cells from the maternal tumour enjoy the benefits of this state and can become implanted in the tissues of the child where they come to be recognized as 'self'. The trophoblast, from which hydatidiform moles and choriocarcinomata develop, is a specialized foetal tissue which is normally in close contact with maternal cells and in which there is a protective mechanism comprising an extra cellular layer of immunologically inert material which separates the foetal cells from the maternal immunocytes. The recipient of a graft of tissue is deliberately treated so as to reduce his immunological competence in order that the grafted organ may survive and function. The reduction in immunological capacity also allows the neoplastic cells to proliferate.

In experimental animals transplantation of tumours from one individual to another, often over many serial passages, is a commonplace. This phenomenon, in sharp contrast to the position in man, may be due to one of three mechanisms. Many laboratory experiments are based on strains of animals which are highly inbred, so that all members of the population carry an almost identical set of genes. In such a syngeneic population all individuals are in almost the same position as a pair of monozygous twins, between whom tissues may be grafted at will. Secondly, in animal work tumours may be selected for their capacity to survive after transplantation and strains of tumour cells of low antigenic potency may be derived. Thirdly, many experimental tumours are virus induced and some transplantation experiments have been equivalent to inoculation of virus contained within living cells.

A reaction of the host to the tumour is seen in many human neoplasms. This consists, first, of a cellular infiltration with lymphocytes and plasma cells and in some cases giant cells of the foreign-body type, and, secondly, of the development of an excess of fibrous tissue. The cellular reaction is particularly prominent in seminoma of the testis and is almost a diagnostic histological feature of this neoplasm. The relationship of the host reaction to the clinical course of the disease has been studied in the case of carcinoma of the breast, the stomach, and the lung, and it has been found that the presence of an active host reaction can be correlated with an increased chance of survival. In addition, it has been found that a reaction in the sinusoids of lymph-nodes not invaded by tumour is of good prognostic significance. This type of investigation is at present in its infancy, and it may be that in the future a detailed histological analysis of the tissues surrounding a tumour may be of value in assessing prognosis and in determining the best line of treatment.

THE ROLE OF IMMUNITY IN THE DEVELOPMENT OF TUMOURS

In this section will be considered the development of tumours as indicative of the formation of masses of neoplastic cells big enough to be seen and to be capable of being identified and in due course capable of extending and of producing fatal disease. This view is to be contrasted with that in CHAPTER VIII which was concerned much more with the changes in cells which lead to their development of a malignant potential.

Several sets of data both on human experience and on investigations in laboratory animals are available which help to throw light on the role of immunological mechanisms in the development of tumours. Tumours are more common in individuals who have an impaired immunological capacity. This is true of humans who suffer from one of the inherited defects of immune capacity and are deficient in either humoral or more particularly cell-mediated immunity.

Careful follow-up studies on patients who have received transplants of organs and have been treated for several years with immunosuppressive drugs have shown that the risk of tumour development is at least one hundred times that in the general population. The risk of tumour development is also higher in animals which have been subjected to thymectomy in early life, and in animals suffering the graft versus host runt disease when reticulo-endothelial cells from an adult have been transplanted early in life.

It has been reported that the frequency of malignant tumours is higher in individuals who have been subjected to tonsillectomy or appendicectomy, and it has been suggested that these operations may have reduced the local defences of the pharynx and of the abdomen. Multiple malignancy, the development of more than one distinct type of malignant neoplasm in a patient either both at the same time or after a time interval, is more often seen with one member of the pair being a reticulo-endothelial tumour affecting the immune system directly than would be expected on the basis of a chance association. Evidence of reduced immunological capacity, especially of the delayed skin-sensitivity type which is a cell-mediated form of immunity, has been found in a series of patients suffering from malignant disease, but whether this is a result of the existing neoplasm or is a causative factor is uncertain. It has also been noted that the increase in the incidence of leukaemia in children, which has been observed over the past two or three decades, has been associated with a concomitant fall in the frequency of death from infection in childhood, and it has been suggested that the children who now develop leukaemia would, in former years, have been liable to die of infection, because of a poorer immunological capacity. Finally, there is a marked difference in tumour incidence between males and females, which cannot be satisfactorily explained on the basis of differences in the environment of the two sexes. The X chromosome carries genes which are responsible for some of the activities of the immune system, and it might be suggested that the female, who has two such chromosomes, might be less likely than the male to develop immunological deficiency. The auto-immune diseases, in which it is postulated that a positive change in the immune system occurs, are more common in females than in males.

This extensive list of observations indicates that the mechanisms of immunity and especially of cellular immunity play a part in the development of neoplastic disease. If it is proved that the immune lymphocytes are important factors in tissue homeostasis, then it can be inferred that anomalies of this system may lead to tumour formation. The evidence in favour of this theory is, however, largely based on the assumption that failure of this mechanism leads to tumour formation, and until further evidence outside the field of tumour pathology is produced, it must be regarded as doubtful. A second possibility is that the mechanism of cell-mediated immunity is capable of destroying some tumour cells, especially those in the circulation, and that the development of a clinically evident neoplasm depends on changes occurring in the cells which eventually become neoplastic and also on a failure of the immune system to recognize such cells as 'not self' and to destroy them.

This second suggestion is attractive because it can be invoked to explain many facets of general tumour pathology. Gradual failure of immunological capacity with advancing age would help to explain the higher frequency of such disease in older people, and the occasional regression of patently malignant tumours and the relatively frequent regression of carcinoma-in-situ may be due to destruction of the abnormal cells by a normal defence mechanism. Studies of venous blood samples from tumour sites have shown that tumour cells are commonly released into the circulation, and follow-up studies have shown that such release is not invariably followed by widespread metastasis. Similarly, it has been shown that if block dissection of the neck is carried out in cases of thyroid carcinoma, small deposits of tumour cells are found in the lymph-nodes in a high proportion of cases. In other series, however, where extensive lymph-node dissection has not been performed, many patients have apparently been cured, although it may be presumed that metastases were present in the lymph-nodes of many of them.

I think it probable that in the course of life many individual cells undergo changes in the genetic structure which release them from the normal controlling factors of tissue homeostasis and that in most instances the abnormal cells are recognized as foreign by the cells of the reticulo-endothelial system and are destroyed, and that for the development of a clinically significant neoplasm it is necessary that this immunological mechanism should break down either because of failure of the immunity cells or because neoplastic cells without foreign surface antigens develop. The system of cell-mediated immunity is most active in the immunological situations in which entire foreign cells are introduced to the body. This is an unusual event in nature and it has been suggested that cell-mediated immunity, which is seen only in higher animals, has evolved not as a defence mechanism against cells gaining entrance to the body from outside but as a defence against intrinsic neoplastic cell transformation. True tumours are almost entirely confined to vertebrates, which also are the group of animals which have developed cell-mediated immunity.

IMMUNOTHERAPY

The ultimate aim of the doctor in studying and trying to understand the phenomena of disease is that he should be able to use the knowledge acquired in prevention of disease and in the treatment of his patients. Immunological techniques may be used in three ways in the treatment of neoplastic disease.

Attempts have been made to increase the level of immunological responsiveness in the individual host by non-specific immunization with BCG, with *Corynebacterium parvum*, and with extracts of yeast cells. Some success has been achieved in experimental animals in which the frequency of induced tumours has been reduced and the progress of developed tumours has been slowed.

Active immunization with malignant cells is equivalent to metastasis and is not helpful in inducing immunity, but tumour cells can be treated by radiation *in vitro* so as to render them inviable, but still antigenically active. Such cells, when injected into an animal with an adjuvant and followed by challenge with transplantable malignant cells, induce a relative immunity to the transplanted neoplastic cells. Some benefit may also be obtained by removing part of a tumour, and, after irradiation *in vitro*, using cells from the original lesion to stimulate immunity.

Passive immunity to tumour cells may be transmitted by the injection of serum from an animal which is showing a response to a neoplasm or which has been immunized by inviable tumour cells or by transplanting lymphocytes or bone-marrow from such an animal to a new host. Cellular passive immunity is a more effective means of increasing the defence of the recipient animal against future challenge with viable malignant cells.

In the human, the clinical response to trials of immunological treatment has been disappointing. This is partly because ethical considerations preclude the use of such methods except in patients for whom the existing methods of therapy have little to offer, which means in general patients with widespread disease whose natural defences are already severely impaired or overcome. Attempts to increase a natural, general, immunological responsiveness meet with little success, and active immunization is similarly attempted in a patient of low potential. A further possible difficulty is that the large mass of cells in a primary tumour and in the secondary deposits may be sufficient to take up all the humoral antibodies and to overwhelm the available cellular defences. Passive immunization in the human in turn produces problems which are not seen in suitably designed animal experiments. Tumours in different human individuals are separate tumours of different antigenic type, and even attempts to induce active immunity in a volunteer host may only give rise to transplantation antibodies which would have adverse effects on the original patient if they were transferred to him, and active lymphoid cells, whether from an immunized donor or from a normal individual, would similarly react with all the tissues of the new host.

CHAPTER XIV

THE PATHOLOGICAL BASIS OF THE CHEMOTHERAPY OF TUMOURS

THE treatment of patients suffering from tumours falls into three distinct modes—surgery, radiation, and chemotherapy—which may be used in combination. It is unnecessary to devote a great deal of space to the pathological bases of the first two forms of treatment. The surgeon is concerned if he can to remove all the tumour which is present, having regard to the mode of extension of the malignant cells by the blood-stream and lymphatics, and the necessity to avoid damage to vital structures, and to avoid unacceptable morbidity. Similarly the radiotherapeutic approach is to attempt to kill tumour cells without damaging the normal cells of surrounding structures, and a number of techniques of fractionated doses and carefully planned direction of radiation have been evolved. The observation that neoplastic cells are more radiosensitive in an environment rich in oxygen has led to the use of hyperbaric oxygen chambers for radiotherapy, and in rare instances, such as that of an iodine-concentrating thyroid tumour, radioactive isotopes selectively taken up by tumour tissue have been used.

The field of chemotherapy, which initially developed on a somewhat empirical basis, has come to be resolved into a series of attempts to interfere selectively with the metabolism of tumour cells, especially with the metabolism and function of the genetic material of those cells. It must be remembered, however, that there are no metabolic pathways specific to neoplastic cells, and, in particular, no specific pathways which are seen in all malignant cells, so that in general chemotherapeutic agents also interfere with the growth and development of normal cells. It is necessary, therefore, in planning and controlling chemotherapy, to recognize that normal components of the body may be adversely affected by the drugs used. These adverse effects are seen most clearly in the haemopoietic system and most drugs used in the therapy of tumours cause depression of the formation of erythrocytes, white blood-cells, and blood platelets, as well as impairment of the immunological defence mechanisms of the body. These adverse side-effects make it necessary to control treatment carefully by observation of the peripheral blood, and also increase the risk of intercurrent infection, so that elaborate aseptic precautions are necessary if intensive therapy is undertaken.

As is so often seen in a study of tumour pathology, the adaptive capacity of tumour cells is important. In many cases remissions have been obtained by chemotherapy but when relapse occurs the tumour cells are resistant to the original drug. To some extent this difficulty can be overcome by using a series of these drugs in a sequential manner and by such methods it is often possible to maintain life in a child with acute leukaemia for two or three years. An alternative approach has been to use a number of drugs in combination in order to attack the neoplastic cells simultaneously from several directions.

The general effects of antitumour drugs may be reduced to some extent by local treatment. This is feasible when a tumour lies within the area of distribution of one major artery, when the drug can be given by intra-arterial injection, and the greater part of its effect will be in the desired area of tumour. This local approach to chemotherapy is showing encouraging results in the treatment of limb tumours and tumours of the central nervous system.

The chemical agents used in the treatment of tumours fall into two major classes, the alkylating agents and antimetabolites, to which must be added a miscellaneous group of substances which, as yet, are not readily grouped. In addition the adrenal corticosteroids have antineoplastic action (*Table IV*).

CORTICOSTEROIDS

Steroid hormones from the adrenal cortex in large doses have an effect on the malignant cells of acute leukaemia and frequently produce a remission in this condition. The mechanism by which this occurs is probably related to a general effect on the metabolism of the body, rather than a specific cytotoxic effect on the cells of the tumour. The general effect of corticosteroids is also valuable in patients with intracranial tumours. When a tumour is present in the cerebrum there is interference with the venous drainage within the head, and oedema, especially around the tumour, is an important cause of loss of cerebral function and of symptoms. The exhibition of corticosteroids acts non-specifically by reducing the oedema with consequent improvement in the clinical condition of the patient. This improvement is non-specific and is not related to the destruction of tumour cells, but it can result in the patient becoming fit for operative and radiotherapeutic procedures.

ALKYLATING AGENTS

Currently the most useful group of chemotherapeutic substances in the treatment of neoplastic diseases is the alkylating agents. These are substances which have two reactive alkyl groups in the molecule and the mode of action is that reactions occur between the alkyl groups and the guanine bases of the DNA helix. These combinations freeze the DNA

Table IV.—DRUGS IN THE TREATMENT OF TUMOURS

Steroids		Acute leukaemia
		Reduction of oedema in brain tumours
Alkylating agents		
Nitrogen mustards	Cyclophosphamide	Hodgkin's disease
		Myeloma
		Chronic lymphatic leukaemia
		Reticulum-cell sarcoma
		Carcinoma of breast and ovary
	Mustine	Hodgkin's disease
		Lymphosarcoma
	Chlorambucil	Chronic lymphatic leukaemia
		Lymphosarcoma
		Hodgkin's disease
		Seminoma
		Carcinoma of breast and ovary
	Mephalan	Myeloma
Dimethane sulphonates	Busulphan	Chronic myeloid leukaemia
Antimetabolites		
Folic acid antagonists	Methotrexate	Acute leukaemia
		Choriocarcinoma
		Burkitt's tumour
Purine antagonists	6-Mercaptopurine ⎫	
	6-Thioguanine ⎬	Acute leukaemia
	Azoguanine ⎭	
Pyrimidine antagonists	5-Fluorouracil ⎫	Acute leukaemia
	6-Azauracil ⎬	Carcinoma of breast
	Cytosine arabinoside ⎭	
	? Urethane	Chronic myeloid leukaemia
Miscellaneous		
Vegetable compounds	Colcemid	Chronic myeloid leukaemia
	Vinblastine	Hodgkin's disease
		Choriocarcinoma
	Vincristine	Acute lymphatic leukaemia
		Reticulum-cell sarcoma
		Hodgkin's disease
Antibiotics	Actinomycin D	Wilms's tumour
		Choriocarcinoma
		Rhabdomyosarcoma
	Mitomycin C	Chronic myeloid leukaemia
		Gastro-intestinal carcinoma
	Mithramycin	Embryonal carcinoma of testis
	Daunorubicin	Acute myeloid leukaemia
L-Asparaginase		Acute leukaemia
		Lymphosarcoma
Methyl aryl hydrazine		Hodgkin's disease
		Reticulum-cell sarcoma
		Melanoma

chain and inhibit uncoiling and replication of the DNA which is an essential preliminary to cell division.

These drugs are of the greatest value in the primary treatment of the diffuse neoplasms of the reticulo-endothelial system, Burkitt's tumour, leukaemia, polycythaemia, Hodgkin's disease, lymphosarcoma,

Alkylating agents

$$RN\begin{cases}CH_2CH_2Cl\\CH_2CH_2Cl\end{cases}$$

$$CH_2\begin{cases}CH_2-NH\\CH_2-O\end{cases}P-N\begin{cases}CH_2CH_2Cl\\CH_2CH_2Cl\end{cases}$$
$$\|$$
$$O$$

Cyclophosphamide

reticulum-cell sarcoma, and myeloma, in which, because of the spread of the disease throughout the body, surgical and radiotherapeutic procedures are less feasible.

Alkylating agents also have an important place in the treatment of tumours which have extended and are no longer susceptible to excision. Encouraging results have been reported in the treatment of solid tumours of the breast, uterus, ovary, bladder, lung, kidney, testis, skin, and the gastro-intestinal tract.

ANTIMETABOLITES

Cell division depends on the duplication of the genetic material of the cell nucleus, DNA, which occurs in the resting nucleus and is a necessary precursor of mitosis. DNA replication in tumour cells depends on the supply of raw materials, in particular the bases adenine, guanine,

Folic acid

Methotrexate

thymidine, and cytosine, which in their sequences comprise the genetic code. Folic acid, after reduction to tetrahydrofolic acid, acts as a co-enzyme in the formation of thymidylic acid, a precursor of thymidine. Methotrexate acts as an antagonist to folic acid because it has a much greater affinity for the reducing enzyme and it thus interferes with the production of the essential base thymidine. Similar competition for enzyme activity is shown by the purine antagonists, 6-mercaptopurine, thioguanine, and azoguanine which interfere with the formation of

Guanine   6 Mercaptopurine

adenine and guanine, and the pyrimidine antagonists, 5-fluorouracil and 6-azauracil, and possibly urethane, which interfere with the production of thymidine and cytosine.

Urical   5 Fluorouracil

The antimetabolites are of value in the treatment of reticulo-endothelial tumours, particularly acute leukaemia, but the most striking therapeutic use of these substances is in the treatment of choriocarcinoma which is a highly malignant neoplasm of foetal tissues occurring in the mother and which is often curable by treatment with methotrexate. A similar striking effect is observed in the lymphoid tumour of children seen mainly in the African continent, Burkitt's lymphoma, which may be cured by very small doses of methotrexate.

MISCELLANEOUS SUBSTANCES

VEGETABLE COMPOUNDS

Colchicine is a substance extracted from the crocus which causes the arrest of mitosis in metaphase. It is widely used for this purpose in laboratory cytological investigation but is too toxic for therapeutic use. A derivative, colcemid, is sometimes used in chronic myeloid leukaemia and Hodgkin's disease. The other two vegetable alkaloids, vinblastine and vincristine, are extracted from a species of periwinkle and both also cause arrest of mitosis in metaphase. Vincristine is currently used in the treatment of acute leukaemia.

PATHOLOGICAL BASIS

ANTIBIOTICS

Four substances produced by micro-organisms of the *Streptomyces* group have useful antineoplastic activity, without undue toxicity. These are actinomycin D, mitomycin C, mithramycin, and daunorubicin. All four form linkages with intranuclear DNA and inhibit the replication of the genetic material or interfere with the function and essential metabolism of cells by preventing the synthesis of RNA and thence of proteins. These compounds are of value in the treatment of acute and chronic myeloid leukaemia and also of the solid tumours, nephroblastoma (Wilms's tumour), choriocarcinoma, embryonal carcinoma of the testis, and some forms of gastro-intestinal cancer.

ASPARAGINASE

Some years ago it was noted that the guinea-pig serum when injected into tumour-bearing animals had an inhibiting effect on the tumours; this was eventually found to be due to the presence of the enzyme asparaginase. The rationale of treatment is that many tumour cells lack the ability to form asparagine and by deamination aspartic acid which is necessary for protein synthesis. Such cells require a supply of preformed asparagine or aspartic acid which is cut off if the enzyme, obtained from guinea-pig serum or from certain strains of *Esch. coli*, is administered, and the growth of the malignant cells is selectively inhibited. Trials of this substance in the treatment of acute leukaemia are currently in progress.

METHYL ARYL HYDRAZINES

These substances act on the mitotic cycle and also induce a high proportion of chromatid breaks, but the mechanism by which this effect is achieved is unknown. They have been useful in the treatment

$$CH_3NHNHCH_2-C_6H_4-CONHCH(CH_3)_2$$

Methyl aryl hydrazine

of Hodgkin's disease and reticulum-cell sarcoma and, rarely, in disseminated malignant melanoma.

I.C.R.F. 159

The most recently described antineoplastic agent is related chemically to the chelating agent ethylene diamine tetra-acetic acid, and in experimental animals has the property of reducing metastases by stimulating the growth of well-formed blood-vessels in the stroma of a tumour and thereby reducing the chance of cells reaching the blood-stream. It is also possible that the action of this agent may depend on an effect on the blood-clotting mechanism, as it has been found that some anticoagulants tend to inhibit neoplastic spread.

CHAPTER XV
TERATOMATA

THE teratomata, etymologically the 'monstrous tumours', form a small group of lesions which are unique in tumour pathology, in that they comprise an assemblage of tissues foreign to the part in which they arise. In a typical teratoma the embryology of the tissues which are seen can be traced to all three of the germ layers of the developing embryo. Skin and nervous tissue from the ectoderm, intestinal and glandular epithelium from the endoderm, and fibrous tissue, bone, and muscle from the mesoderm can all be identified in the substance of one tumour. This is in contrast to the mixed tumours mentioned in CHAPTERS II and V, where a collection of tissues derived from one germ layer, the mesoderm, are seen together.

The commonest site for teratoma is the ovary, where the lesion is usually benign and cystic, commonly contains hairs and teeth, and is lined by stratified squamous epithelium. This tumour, the dermoid cyst, outnumbers all other forms of teratoma. After the ovary, the commonest site is the testis, where the lesion is most often malignant. These two sites comprise the gonads in the two sexes; other sites are less frequent and include the sacrococcygeal region, the anterior mediastinum, the thyroid region of the neck, the retroperitoneum, and the central nervous system, usually close to the pineal body. The sites of origin of these lesions can be divided into two. The first group comprises the gonads, and the retroperitoneal sites at which germ cells may be sequestrated during their path from the yolk sac to the urogenital ridge and thence caudally, as the definitive gonad assumes its final position. Secondly, there are midline situations where the neuroectodermal groove has closed or where the investing ectoderm has joined anteriorly to enclose the body of the embryo.

Teratomata, like other tumours, may be benign or malignant. Most testicular teratomata are malignant, most others are benign, although teratomata of the sacrococcygeal region, if left in situ, will almost inevitably develop an aggressive or malignant character. Two modes of expression of malignancy are seen in teratomata. The whole lesion may have a malignant potential and the metastases consist of a conglomeration of tissues similar to that seen in the primary tumour (*Fig.* 13). Less commonly a malignant neoplasm may develop in one of the differentiated tissues and then behave as a carcinoma, sarcoma, melanoma, or carcinoid according to its origin. It is, however, unwise to invoke one-sided development of a teratoma to explain an unusual tumour unless there is positive evidence of a teratomatous origin.

Detailed histological examination of the structure of teratomata shows that not only do they comprise cells which can be identified as belonging to the several tissues of the body, of different germ-layer origin, but that these are arranged in an organoid pattern. Epithelium of respiratory type is seen in tubules which are surrounded by fibrous tissue and smooth muscle, and which have in the walls plaques of cartilage similar to those in the walls of bronchi. Squamous epithelium is found with skin appendages, sweat-glands, sebaceous glands, and hair follicles. Bone and cartilage are found together and occasionally the anlage of a joint with two fragments of bone capped by cartilage and separated by a synovial space can be identified (*Figs.* 14, 15, 16). In very rare instances an even greater degree of organoid differentiation can be found, digits and parts of limbs have been recognized, and in one or two instances a short axial skeleton. The organoid differentiation is not always adult in type. A few tumours of the ovary and of the testis have been described in which there were structures closely resembling the entire presomite embryo. This capacity for a wide range of organoid differentiation appears to be inherent in the teratoma cell. Individual cells from animal teratomata have been shown to have the capacity, on transplantation, of growing into tumour masses containing a wide variety of tissue elements. The peculiar histological appearance of the teratoma indicates that the cells which comprise the tumour are capable of the full range of differentiative capacity and are also able to influence each other's development, most probably by the action of a system of organizers analogous to that which develops in the embryo and leads to the normal co-ordinated development of the fully formed human.

A further microscopic peculiarity of these tumours is that some teratomata in males contain sex chromatin particles. It became possible in 1949 to determine the sex of an individual of some species including the human by examination of the nuclei of somatic cells. The sex chromatin particle, the Barr body, is a small dense mass of condensed chromatin which is seen lying close to the nuclear membrane in a high proportion of the cells of females, but is not seen in the cells of males. It is believed that this particle comprises the inactivated second X chromosome of the female and that it is not seen in the male because the male sex chromosome constitution is XY, and the genes located on this single X chromosome are necessary for normal cell function, and that therefore this single X chromosome is not inactivated and condensed. This sex chromatin particle has been identified with certainty in the cells of testicular teratomata by many workers, but its presence in other teratomata of males is doubtful. It has been shown that the chromosome constitution of the hosts of testicular teratomata is normal. Unfortunately, chromosome analysis has not helped in the identification of these lesions, as the cells which can be cultivated from testicular teratomata are usually aneuploid and an accurate assessment of the chromosome constitution cannot be made.

The interesting problem posed by the teratomata is that of their origin. Any hypothesis of the origin of these tumours must account for the wide range of cellular differentiation, for the presence of organoid differentiation, for the predilection for the gonads, and for midline sites, and for the presence of sex chromatin in the tumours of males. I have discussed in CHAPTER V the problems of differentiation in tumours, and have indicated that, in general, the cells of any situation of the body have only a limited capacity for differentiation along one line, that it is as if some of the genetic capacity of the cells was permanently blocked. This implies that some mode of origin other than that involved for the generality of tumours is necessary. Three major hypotheses have been put forward.

The first is that teratomata represent included twins. The pregnancy which resulted in the host of the tumour was a twin pregnancy in which one member was abnormal in form and was included within the body of the other. This suggestion would conveniently explain the teratomata which arise in the sacrococcygeal region, the mediastinum, the head, and the abdomen which are all sites at which conjoined, Siamese, twins are attached, but does not explain the large number of gonadal teratomata. Furthermore, this suggestion does not provide a satisfactory explanation for the presence of sex chromatin in testicular teratomata. If it is assumed that the foetus is capable of developing immunological tolerance to implanted foreign cells such as those of a twin, it could be suggested that the teratomata of males might include tissues from female twins; however, the reverse situation, which should be equally likely, does not occur. Teratomata in females with a male nuclear pattern are not seen, and in the recorded cases of conjoined twins both have been found to be of the same sex.

A second hypothesis is that teratomata arise from rests of totipotent cells which have escaped the action of primary or secondary organizers and are able to show the full range of genetic capacity of the human cell. This attractive hypothesis does not explain the distribution of the sites of these tumours, nor does it offer an explanation of the presence of sex chromatin in testicular teratomata.

The third suggestion is that teratomata arise by the parthenogenetic development of germ cells. The germ cells, oogonia and spermatogonia, have the function of carrying genetic material from the parents to the new zygote and, after fusion, produce a cell which has, almost by definition, the full capacity to develop into a complete individual. In the course of their life cycle the germ cells undergo a specialized form of division, reduction division, or meiosis, which results in the formation of haploid cells each containing half the normal chromosome number. If two haploid cells fuse, the result is a diploid cell which could have the genetic potential of a zygote. In the case of the female all haploid cells contain one X chromosome, and, after fusion, the diploid cell will contain two X chromosomes, the normal female complement. In the male, on the other hand, half the haploid cells will contain an X chromosome and half will contain a Y chromosome. Fusion of two haploid cells will produce diploid cells of the constitution XX, XY, or YY and the first of these may be expected to show a sex chromatin particle. This hypothesis explains the common gonadal site of teratomata and the presence of sex chromatin in testicular tumours of this type. The occasional retroperitoneal teratomata can be regarded as taking origin from germ cells sequestered during their migration across the abdomen, but it is difficult to invoke this hypothesis for the teratomatous tumours of the mediastinum or the brain.

Some help in deciding among these suggestions may be obtained from clinical considerations. Teratomata of the ovary and of the testis are most often seen in adults in whom the changes of puberty and activation of the germ cells have occurred. Sacrococcygeal teratomata, on the other hand, are almost invariably seen soon after birth and intracranial and mediastinal teratomata are usually evident in young individuals.

The problem of the origin of these curious lesions can best be solved by postulating two modes of origin. I suggest that the gonadal teratomata, and possibly those of the posterior abdominal wall, are of germ-cell origin, and that they arise by parthenogenetic development of haploid germ cells, while the extragonadal teratomata, for the most part, take origin from cells at the edges of the embryonic disk which have escaped organization. An exceedingly rare example of the latter type is the teratoma-like mass of tissue which is seen in the umbilical cord or in the placenta. It is a matter of semantics rather than of pathology, whether these lesions are regarded as included twins or not. Identical twins are formed by the separation of groups of cells at a very early stage in embryogenesis, conjoined twins, in which both individuals are more or less fully formed, derive from an incomplete separation. The line of demarcation between a malformed conjoined twin and a teratoma may be very indistinct indeed. I feel that this dual hypothesis of the origin of teratomata explains the observed data in this group of lesions, and that it may help in understanding their clinical manifestations. I hope that it may lead to further studies which will add to our understanding.

FURTHER READING

Detailed documentation by references to original work is inappropriate in a book of this kind which is intended as an introduction to the subject rather than as a definitive work of reference. Further information and references can be obtained from the section on general pathology in any good systematic text such as that of Anderson, and a list of useful monographs is appended. This field of study is continually expanding and articles dealing with the general pathology of tumours are to be found throughout the medical literature, especially in the journals *Cancer, The British Journal of Cancer, The Journal of the National Cancer Institute, The European Journal of Cancer, The International Journal of Cancer*, and *Cancer Research*.

AMBROSE, E. J., and ROE, F. J. C. (eds.) (1966), *The Biology of Cancer*. London: Van Nostrand.
ANDERSON, W. A. D. (ed.) (1966), *Pathology*, 5th ed. St. Louis: Mosby.
BOESEN, E., and DAVIS, W. (1970), *Cytotoxic Drugs in the Treatment of Cancer*. London: Arnold.
BRAIN, LORD (1963), 'The Neurological Complications of Neoplasms', *Lancet*, **1**, 179.
BRAUN, A. C. (1969), *The Cancer Problem*. New York: Columbia University Press.
BURNET, F. M. (1969), *Self and Non Self*. Cambridge: Cambridge University Press.
— — (1970), *Immunological Surveillance*. London: Pergamon.
EVANS, R. W. (1966), *The Histological Appearances of Tumours*, 2nd ed. Edinburgh: Livingstone.
FOULDS, L. (1969), *Neoplastic Development*, Vol. 1. London: Academic Press.
FRY, R. J. M., GRIEM, M. L., and KIRSTEN, W. H. (eds.) (1969), *Normal and Malignant Cell Growth. Recent Results in Cancer Research*, No. 17. Heidelberg: Springer-Verlag.
GROSS, L. (1970), *Oncogenic Viruses*, 2nd ed. London: Pergamon.
LYNCH, H. T. (1967), *Heredity Factors in Carcinoma. Recent Results in Cancer Research*, No. 12. Heidelberg: Springer-Verlag.
RAVEN, R. W., and ROE, F. J. C. (eds.) (1967), *The Prevention of Cancer*. London: Butterworths.
RUSSFIELD, A. B. (1966), *Tumors of Endocrine Glands and Secondary Sex Organs*. U.S. Public Health Service Publication No. 1332. Washington, D.C., U.S.A.
SCOTT, R. B. (1970), 'Cancer Chemotherapy—the First Twenty-five Years', *Br. med. J.*, **4**, 259.
SMITHERS, D. W. (1964), *On the Nature of Neoplasia in Man*. Edinburgh: Livingstone.
TURK, J. L. (1969), *Immunology in Clinical Medicine*. London: Heinemann.
WHITEHOUSE, H. L. K. (1965), *Towards an Understanding of the Mechanism of Heredity*. London: Arnold.
WILLIS, R. A. (1952), *The Spread of Tumours in the Human Body*, 2nd ed. London: Butterworths.
— — (1968), *Pathology of Tumours*, 4th ed. London: Butterworths.

INDEX

	PAGE
ABDOMINAL skin cancer(s) due to heat	56
— — — in mule spinners	60
Aberrant differentiation	30
— hormone production by tumours	16, 80
Acanthosis nigricans associated with gastro-intestinal cancer	17
Acoustic neuroma, bilateral	48
Acromegaly	74
Addison's disease due to adrenal gland tumours	82
Adenoma malignum (*Fig.* 8)	33, 34, 45
Adenomatosis, pluriglandular	80
Adrenal cortex, tumours of	75
— glands, hormones of	75
— medulla, tumours of	76
— tumours causing Addison's disease	82
Adrenaline	76
Adrenocorticotrophic hormone, excess of	74
— — production by tumours	81
Aflatoxin causing cancer	62
Agammaglobulinaemia, tumour formation associated with	52
Age, incidence of tumour in relation to	45
Alcohol, carcinoma associated with high intake of	61
Aldosterone secretion, excessive	75
Alkylating agents	61, 93
Allergic reaction to tumour	17, 18
Alpha-fetoglobulin in blood in presence of liver cancer	86
Anabolic steroids in treatment of tumours	84
Androgenic hormones in treatment of tumours	84
Angiofibroma	29
Animal(s) experiments, interpretation of results in terms of human pathology	59
— viral oncogenesis in	65
Antibiotics	94, 97
Antibodies, system of humoral	85
Antibody-producing cells	85
Antidiuretic hormone	74
— — production by tumours	81
Antigens	85
— of tumour cells	86

	PAGE
Antimetabolites	93, 95
Antitumour drugs	93
Appendix, carcinoid tumour of	78
Argentaffin tissues, carcinoid tumours of	7, 8
Argentaffin-cell tumours causing endocrine activity	16
Arrhenoblastoma	78
Arsenic as carcinogen	62
Asbestos as carcinogen	61, 63
Asparaginase	94, 97
Atomic energy, increased risk of neoplastic disease due to work on	57
Auricle, myxoma of	13
Auto-immune diseases	85, 86, 89
Azauracil, 6-	94, 96
Azo-compounds	61
Azoguanine	94, 96
BARR body in testicular teratomata	99
Basal-cell carcinoma of skin (*Figs.* 2–4)	5, 7
— naevus	49
Benign teratoma	98
— tumour(s), normal chromosome content of cells of	53
— — and malignant (*Fig.* 1)	4
— — — change in	33
— — spread of	19
Beryllium as carcinogen	62
Bile-duct(s) obstruction by tumour	13, 14
— spread of metastases by	20, 23
Bladder cancer associated with schistosomiasis	56
— — association between smoking and	62
— — as occupational hazard	63
— mixed tumour of	29, 30
— papilloma	6
— — malignant change in	33
— spread of metastases along	20, 23
Bladder-wall metastases	23
Blood group A, association of gastric cancer with	52
Blood-borne metastases	20, 21
Blood-vessels, effects of tumour on	12
— malignant tumours invading	21
Blue-rubber bleb naevus	49

INDEX

Bone cancer due to radioactive strontium .. 58
— metastases .. 20
— sarcoma due to ingestion of luminous paint .. 57
— tumours .. 8
— — giant-cell .. 7
Bone-marrow, metastases in .. 20
— secondaries in .. 12
— tumour causing anaemia .. 15
Bowen's disease .. 32
Brain, teratoma of .. 101
— tumour causing hydrocephalus 13
— — corticosteroid therapy in 84, 93
— — variation of histological structure in large .. 39
Breast adenocarcinoma, precursor of 33
— cancer, hormonal cause of .. 83
— — hormone-dependent .. 83
— — hormones and endocrine gland ablation in treatment of 83, 84
— — spread of .. 19
— intraduct carcinoma of, malignant change in .. 33
— mixed tumour of .. 30
— osteosarcoma .. 31
Bronchi, obstruction of, by tumour 14
Bronchial adenoma .. 16
— — carcinoid .. 78
— carcinoma, squamous .. 34
— hamartoma .. 7, 30
Burkitt's lymphoma, chemotherapy in .. 94, 96
— — regression of .. 41
— — and sickle-cell disease 52, 69
— — viral aetiology of .. 68
Busulphan .. 94

CABLE workers, bladder cancer in .. 63
Café-au-lait spots of Peutz-Jegher syndrome .. 17
Calcitonin .. 74
Calcium, excess of, in urine, in parathyroid tumour .. 76
'Cancer families' .. 52
Carcinogenesis, two-stage mechanism of .. 44
Carcinogenic substances .. 58
Carcinogens, elemental .. 62
— environmental .. 55
Carcinoid syndrome .. 78
— tumours of argentaffin tissues .. 7, 8
Carcinoma (see also under specific parts and types)
— histology of .. 28
Carcinoma-in-situ .. (Fig. 7) 5, 32
— of cervix .. (Fig. 7) 33
— — treatment .. 37
— histological entity .. 35
Carcinomatous neuropathy .. 18

Carcinosarcoma .. (Fig. 6) 9, 30
Cartilaginous hamartoma of bronchus .. 30
Catecholamines, adrenal secretion of 75, 76
Cell(s) differentiation .. 26
— — and tumour formation .. 28
— disorderly proliferation of precancerous .. 33
— division, capacity for .. 27
— — — and tumour formation .. 28
— form and function, range of .. 25
— genome, changes in, due to viral invasion .. 70, 71
— growth, excessive, in tumour .. 3
— — mechanism of control of .. 4
— — uncontrolled, in malignancy 3
— multiplication of viruses in .. 65
— reactions to viral invasion .. 70
Cell-mediated immunity, anomalies of, leading to tumour formation 89
— — system of .. 85
Cellular reaction of host to tumour 87
Cerebral metastases .. 21
— oedema due to brain tumour 13, 93
Cerebrospinal fluid, spread of metastases through .. 23
Cervical cancer, herpes simplex virus and .. 69
— — in parous women .. 83
— — spread of .. 23
— carcinoma, environmental factors concerned in .. 62
— teratoma .. 98
Cervix, carcinoma-in-situ of (Fig. 7) 33
— — treatment .. 37
Chemical carcinogenesis .. 58
— carcinogens and Shope papilloma virus, synergistic action of .. 66
— laboratory staff, bladder cancer in 63
Chemotherapeutic agent, development by tumour of resistance to 39, 47
Chemotherapy, antitumour, side-effects on normal cells .. 92
— of tumours, pathological basis of 92
Children, Africa, Burkitt's lymphoma in .. 68, 69
Chlorambucil .. 94
Chorio-adenoma destruens .. 7, 9
Choriocarcinoma of testis, remission of primary .. 41
Chorionepithelioma .. 9, 78, 96
— malignant, hormone production by .. 73
Chorionic tumours of placenta, endocrine activity of .. 16
Chromium as carcinogen .. 62
Chromophobe adenoma of pituitary causing decreased flow of hormones .. 82

INDEX

	PAGE
Chromosome(s) aberration associated with polycythaemia and myeloid leukaemia	54
— analysis of tumour cells	39
— marker	53
— Philadelphia	54
— and tumours	53
Cigarette smoking as cause of cancer	44, 59, 61
Circumcision in relation to cancer of cervix and of penis	62, 63
Climatic conditions associated with Burkitt's lymphoma	68
Clinicopathological correlation in tumours	11
Coal-miners, health hazards of	64
Co-carcinogens	58
Coelomic surfaces, spread of metastases over	22
Colcemid	94, 96
Colitis, ulcerative, colonic cancer associated with	56
Colon, cancer of, causing obstruction	13
— — embryonic gut antigen in blood in	86
— — prognositic classification	10
— — without polyposis	48
— liver metastases of	21
— polyps of (see Polyposis Coli)	
— in Gardner's syndrome	50
Connective tissue, metaplasia in	27
Connective-tissue abnormalities in tuberose sclerosis	50
— cells, tumour of	28
— tumours	7, 8, 9
— — associated with hypoglycaemia	16
— — of meninges and nerve-sheaths	23
Contraceptives, oral, causing endometrial hyperplasia	83
Corticosteroid(s) as antitumour drugs	93
— treatment of tumours	84
Cortisone and cortisol	75
Cushing's syndrome	74, 75
Cyclophosphamide	94, 95
Cylindromatosis	49
Cyst, dermoid	98
Cystadenocarcinoma of ovary	15
Cytosine arabinoside	94
DEOXYRIBOSENUCLEIC acid (see DNA)	
Dermatomyositis associated with tumour	17
Dermoid cyst	98
Development, normal	26
Diabetes due to pancreatic carcinoma	82
Diaphysial aclasis	32, 37, 49
Diarrhoea due to colonic tumour	12
Differentiation, aberrant	30
— of cells	25, 26

	PAGE
Differentiation, changes in, in progression of tumour (*Figs.* 9–12)	38
— in teratoma (*Figs.* 14–16)	99, 100
— tumours	28
DNA	47
— action of alkylating agents on	93
— of cell nucleus and genetic blocking in cells	27
— mode of action of antimetabolites on	95
— substances inducing chemical changes in bases of	61
— ultra-violet radiation damage to	56
— as viral component	70
Dominant gene, abnormal, leading to tumour formation	49
Dormant cancer cells	24
Down's syndrome, chromosome anomaly in, and leukaemia	54
Drug(s) resistance, rapid build-up of, in tumour cells	93
— used in treatment of tumours	93
Duct, obstruction of, by tumour	13
Dust inhalation causing cancer	64
Dye-stuffs manufacture causing bladder cancer	63
Dysphagia due to mediastinal tumour	14
E.B. VIRUS and Burkitt's lymphoma	69
Electro-encephalographic effects of tumour	12
Elemental carcinogens	62
Embryo, differentiation of cells of	26
Embryonic tumours	7, 8
Endocrine adenomatosis, multiple	49
— deficiency due to tumours	81
— gland ablation in treatment of tumours	83, 84
— hyperplasia, multiple	80
— organs, hormonally active tumours of	73
— — hormone-secreting tumours of	16
— — pituitary control of	73, 74
— — tumours of several	80
— phenomena due to tumours	16
Endometrial hyperplasia (*Fig.* 1)	5
— — due to excessive oestrogens	83
Endometrium, cancer of, hormonal causes of	83
— mixed mesodermal tumour of	9, 30
Energy, apportionment between differentiation and reproduction	27, 29
Environmental factors in tumour formation	55
Enzyme action, deficiency of, in xeroderma pigmentosa	51, 57
Epilepsy due to tumour	12
Epiloia (*see* Tuberose Sclerosis)	

INDEX

	PAGE		PAGE
Epithelial cells, tumour of	28	Genetically determined conditions leading to malignancy	32
— tissue, metaplasia in	27	Genetics and tumours	47
— tumour(s)	8	Genotype interaction with environment to form tumour	47
— — lymphatic spread of	22		
Epithelioma adenoides cysticum	49	Germ cells	77
Evolutionary adaptation of malignant tumour	39, 47	— — parthogenetic development of, as origin of teratoma	100, 101
— — tumour cells	39, 40, 83	Giant-cell epulis	76
		Giant-celled tumours	40
FALLOPIAN tube, passage of cancer cells along	23	Gigantism	74
		Glial cell tumours	8, 30
Feedback, failure of negative, and tumour formation	82	Gliomata, spread of metastases from	23
		Glucagon production	76
Female genital tract, spread of metastases through	20, 23	Gonadal teratomata	98, 99, 101
		— tumours associated with Turner's syndrome	54
Fibro-adenoma of breast	30		
Fibroid of uterus (*see* Uterine Fibroid)		Gonadotrophic hormone	78, 79
Fibrosarcoma in fowls, virus causing	66	Gonadotrophin, chorionic, tumours producing	81
Fistula formation due to tumour	14	Gonads, hormones of	77
Fluorouracil, 5-	94, 96	Granular-cell myoblastoma	7
Foetal dangers in X-ray examination of mother	57	Granulosa-cell tumour of ovary, hormones produced by	78
Foetal-tissue tumours	8, 9	Growth hormone, excess of	74
Foetus, development of tolerance to tissue cells in	85, 87	Gynaecomastia due to tumours of gonadal stroma	77
— transmission of tumours between mother and	87		
Folic acid	95, 96	HAEMOPOIETIC system, effects of antitumour drugs on	92
Food additives causing cancer	62	— tissue tumours	8
		Haemorrhage due to tumour	12
GAMMA-RAYS as cause of cancer	57	Hamartomata	7, 8, 30
Ganglioneuroma, regression of neuroblastoma to	41	Haploid cells, parthenogenetic development of, as cause of teratoma	101
Gardner's syndrome	50		
Gastric carcinoma, association with blood group A	52	Heat, long-continued exposure to, causing skin cancer	56
— — in coal-miners	64	Hepatoblastoma, regression of	41
Gastro-intestinal cancer associated with acanthosis nigricans	17	Herpes labialis, dormant virus of	70
		— simplex virus and cervical cancer	69
— — blood-borne metastases from	21	Hilus-cell tumour of ovary	78
Genes, effect of environment on	51	Histiocytic reticulosis, familial	48
— injury to, from radioactivity and ionizing radiation	58	Hollow viscera, effects of tumour of	13
— single, and tumours	48	Homeostasis, immune processes and	85, 86, 89
— — — of endocrine organs	80	Hormonal activity in non-endocrine tumour cells	31
Genetic activity, controlling mechanism	47	Hormone(s) as aetiological factors in tumours	82
— blocking	27, 28	— produced by tumours	73
— — release of, in tumours	29, 31	— production, aberrant, by tumours	16, 80
— cause(s) of colonic and intestinal polyps	50	— — by tumours of non-endocrine organs	16
— — polyposis coli	45	— in treatment of tumours	83, 84
— material, basic (*see* DNA)		— and tumours	73
— — in cell	25	Hormone-dependent tumours	83
— — — changes in, during differentiation	25	Hydatidiform mole	9, 78
Genetically controlled tumours, single-gene	48	Hydrocarbons, polycyclic	60

106

INDEX

	PAGE
Hydrocephalus due to brain tumour	13
Hydroxytryptamine, 5-, production of	78
Hyperbaric oxygen chamber in radiotherapy to tumour	92
Hypercalcaemia, tumours causing	81
Hyperglycaemia, tumours causing	81
Hypernephroma invading renal vein and inferior vena cava	21
Hyperthyroidism	74
Hypoglycaemia, connective-tissue tumours associated with	16
— due to islet-cell tumours	77
— tumours causing	81
Hypothalamic control of pituitary	73
Humoral antibodies, system of	85
I.C.R.F. 159	97
Immune deficiency, role of oncogenesis	46, 59
— processes, relationship to neoplastic disease	44, 48
Immunity in explanation of regression	41
— role of, in development of tumours	59, 88
— and tumours	85
Immunization, active, with irradiated tumour cells	90
— non-specific, to increase immunological responsiveness	90
— passive	90
Immunoglobulin production	85
Immunological defence, methods of	85
— — system, effect of antitumour drugs on	92
— reaction to tumours	86
— response to antigens	85, 86
Immunosuppression and carcinogenesis	59
— due to tumours	17
Immunosuppressive therapy increasing risk of tumour formation	88
Immunotherapy	90
Infection in presence of tumour	14, 17
— of tumour	14
Inhaled carcinogens	64
Initiating and promoting agents in oncogenesis	44, 58
Injury as factor in tumour formation	55
Insulin excess associated with tumours	81
— production	76
Intestinal obstruction by tumour	14
— polyposis and neurofibromatosis of Peutz-Jegher syndrome	17
— polyps of Peutz-Jegher syndrome	50
— tumour, effects	14
Intra-arterial injection of antitumour drug	93

	PAGE
Intraduct carcinoma of breast, malignant change in	33
Intraluminal tumours causing obstruction	14
Intussusception due to polypoid tumour causing obstruction	14
Ionizing radiation causing cancer	57, 58
Iron as carcinogenic	62
Irradiation as cause of cancer	44, 56
Irritative effects of tumour	12
Islet-cell tumours	77
Isonicotinic acid hydrazide causing cancer	62
KERATOSIS palmaris et plantaris	50
— senile, of skin, malignant change in	33
Kidney tumours, spread of metastases from	23
LABORATORY animals, development of susceptible strains	48
— — inducing tumours in, by hormone administration	82
— — study of viral oncogenesis in	66
— — tumour transplantation in	87
Lactones causing cancer	62
Langerhans, tumours of islets of	77
'Latent' carcinoma of prostate	33, 34
Letterer-Siwe disease	48
Leuco-erythroblastic anaemia due to tumour	12
Leucoplakia	33, 37
Leucosis, avian	65
Leukaemia(s), acute, adaptation of cells in, to environmental changes	39
— — associated with Down's syndrome	54
— — corticosteroid(s) in	93
— — — therapy causing remission in	84
— in cats	65
— cell survival in circulating blood in	24
— deaths of children from, and survival from infections	88
— epidemiological studies	69
— following X-ray therapy	57
— fowls	66
— myeloid, following polycythaemia, chromosome aberration associated with	54
— serial karyotype analyses of cells of	39
— 'virus particles' and mycoplasmata in blood in	69
— in X-ray workers	57

107

INDEX

Leukaemic transformation of bone-marrow due to radioactive strontium 58
Lipoma, enormous 15
Liver cancer, alpha-fetoglobulin in blood in 86
— — spread through bile-ducts .. 23
— metastases 20, 21
— tumour(s) due to aflatoxin .. 62
— — obstructing bile-ducts .. 14
Local effects of tumour 11
— spread of malignant tumour 4, 19
Lung cancer, association between smoking and 62
— — blood-borne metastases from 21
— — cough of 12
— — in coal-miners 64
— — due to radon inhalation .. 57
— — infection complicating .. 14
— — small-cell 29, 31
— — transpleural spread 22
— carcinoma, malignancy of .. 5
— metastases 20
— mixed tumour of 29
— osteosarcoma 31
— tumours, hormone production by 16, 81
Lymph-node metastases .. 20, 22
Lymphatic metastases .. 20, 22
Lymphoma, Burkitt's (*see also* Burkitt's Lymphoma)
— — regression of 41
— in cattle 65

MALABSORPTION due to intestinal tumour 14
Malaria, association of Burkitt's lymphoma with 69
— and sickle-cell disease 53
Malignant change, development of 32
— — in xeroderma pigmentosa 51, 56
— meningitis 23
— teratoma .. .. .. (*Fig.* 13) 98
— tumour(s), abnormal chromosome content of cells of 53
— — and benign tumours (*Fig.* 1) 4
— — conception of, as parasitic entity .. 39, 47, 53, 83
— — local extension of .. 4, 19
— — metastases of .. 4, 19, 20
— — in relation to reduced immunological capacity .. 88
— — spread of 4, 19
— — uncontrolled cell multiplication in 3
Mammary cancer in mice, experimental 66
'Marker chromosomes' 53
Masculinization due to adrenal cortical tumour 75

Masculinization due to ovarian tumour 78
Mediastinal teratoma .. 98, 101
Mediastinum, tumour of, distorting oesophagus 14
Meiosis 101
Meningeal spaces, spread of metastases through .. 20, 23
Meningioma, malignancy of, assessed by chromosome constitution .. 54
Meningitis, malignant 23
Mephalan 94
Mercaptopurine, 6- 94, 96
Mesodermal tumours, mixed 9, 30
Metabolic action of carcinogens .. 59
— effects of tumours 16
Metabolism, hormone control of .. 73
Metaplasia 27
Metastasis(es) 4, 19, 20
— mechanisms of 20
— sites of 20
— of teratoma .. (*Fig.* 13) 98
Metastatic deposits, histological appearances of, and primary tumour 39
Methotrexate 94, 95, 96
Methyl aryl hydrazines .. 94, 97
Milk, transmission of cancer virus in mothers' 67
Mining, health hazards of 64
Mixed tumours .. (*Figs.* 5, 6) 8, 9
— — differentiation in 29
Mongolism (*see* Down's Syndrome)
Multistage hypothesis of oncogenesis 45
Mustine 94
Myasthenia gravis associated with tumour of thymus 16
Mycoplasmata in blood in leukaemia 69
Myeloma, multiple 48
Myoblastoma, granular cell .. 7
Myxoma of auricle 13

NAEVUS, basal-cell 49
— blue-rubber bleb 49
Naphthylamines 61
Neoplastic disease, absence of necessary cause 43
— — definitions 3
Nephroblastoma 48
— regression of 41
Nerve-fibres, over-stimulation of, by tumour 12
Nervous system, central, teratoma of 98, 101
Neuroblastoma of adrenal medulla 76
— regression of, to ganglioneuroma 41
Neurofibromatosis 49
Neuropathy, carcinomatous .. 18
Nickel as carcinogen 62
Nipple, Paget's disease of .. 33, 35, 37
Nitrosamines 61

108

INDEX

	PAGE
Noradrenaline	76
Nuclear devices, increased radiation from fall-out from, hazards	57
OAT-CELL carcinoma of lung, ACTH produced by	81
Occupational cancer hazard	63
Oedema due to brain tumour	13, 93
Oesophageal distortion due to mediastinal tumour	14
Oesophagus, carcinoma of, associated with tylosis	50
Oestrogen excess causing endometrial cancer	83
— — — — hyperplasia	83
— — of, in gonadal tumour	78
— treatment of prostatic cancer	83, 84
— — tumours in postmenopausal women	84
Oncogenesis .. .. .. (*Fig.* 8)	42
— viral (*see* Viral Oncogenesis)	
Organ transplants, immunosuppressive therapy after, and tumour formation	88
Organoid differentiation in teratoma (*Figs.* 14–16)	99, 100
Osteitis fibrosa cystica	76
Osteochondroma	29
Osteoclastoma	7
Osteomyelitis, chronic, skin carcinoma associated with ulcers of	56
Osteosarcoma of lung and breast	31
Ovarian cystadenocarcinoma	15
— metastases	22
— teratoma	98, 101
— — carcinoid	78, 79
— tumours, sexual effects of	77
Ovary, spread of metastases to and from	23
'PAGET cells'	33
Paget's disease of nipple	33, 35, 37
Pain of cancer, mechanism of	12
Pancreas, carcinoma of, causing diabetes	82
— tumour of head of	13
Pancreatic islets, hormones of	76
— tumours, islet-cell, causing Zollinger-Ellison syndrome	77
Pancreatic-duct obstruction by tumour	13
Papillary carcinoma of bladder	6
Papilloma (*see also under specific part*)	
— of bladder, malignant change in	33
— in rabbits, virus causing	66
Paradoxical lymphatic spread of cancer	22
Parahormone, excess of, due to parathyroid tumour	76

	PAGE
Paralysis due to tumour	15
Paralytic ileus due to cancer	13
Parasitic entity, conception of malignant tumour as	39, 47, 53, 83
Parasitization, tumour	15
Parathyroid glands, hormone of	76
Parthenogenetic development of germ cell as cause of teratoma	100, 101
Passenger virus	70
Pathological classification of tumours (*Figs.* 2–6)	6, 7
— fractures due to tumour	15
Pedunculated tumour, vascular obstruction due to torsion of	13
Pelvic metastases	22
— peritoneum metastases in	22
— tumour obstructing ureter	13
Pericardial cavity, spread of metastases across	22
Peritoneal cavity, spread of metastases across	20, 22
— fluid, tumour cell survival in	22
Peutz-Jegher syndrome	32, 50
— — café-au-lait spots of	17
Phaeochromocytoma	7, 48
— associated with medullary carcinoma of thyroid	80
— — — thyroid carcinoma	49
'Philadelphia chromosome'	54
Physical factors in tumour formation	55
Pia arachnoid, tumour cells in	23
Pigmented-cell tumours	8
Pituitary adenoma causing decreased flow of hormones	82
— control of endocrine organs	73, 74
— gland, hormones of	74
— tumour causing gigantism and acromegaly	74
— — effects	16
Placenta, teratoma-like mass in	101
— tumours of	78
Placental barrier, passage of cancer virus across	67
Placental-hormone production by lung tumours	16
Plastic film implants as cause of sarcoma	56
Pleural cavities, spread of metastases across	20, 22
— neoplasms due to asbestos	61, 63
Pluriglandular adenomatosis	80
Pneumonia secondary to lung cancer	14
Polycyclic hydrocarbons	60
Polycythaemia due to renal carcinoma	16
Polygenic factors in tumour formation	51
Polyoma virus	67
Polypoid lesions causing obstruction	14
Polyposis coli	50
— — genetic cause	45

INDEX

	PAGE
Polyposis coli, malignant change in (*Fig.* 8)	32, 33, 34, 37, 45, 51
Polyps of colon (*see* Polyposis Coli)	
— intestinal, of Peutz-Jegher syndrome	32
Porta hepatis, metastases in lymph-nodes of	13
Portal system, spread of metastases by	21
Precancerous state .. (*Figs.* 7, 8)	32
Pregnancy, danger to child of X-ray examination in	57
'Premalignant' component of gene in tylosis	50
Primary tumours, undetectable	24
Primates, study of viral oncogenesis in	67
Progesterone, excess of, in gonadal tumour	78
Prognostic classification of tumours	6, 10
Progression .. .. (*Figs.* 9–12)	38
Promoting and initiating agents in oncogenesis	44, 58
Prostaglandins	79
Prostate, carcinoma of, obstructing urethra	13
— 'latent' carcinoma of	33, 34
— — — histological entity	35, 36
Prostatic cancer, oestrogen treatment of	83, 84
Psychological changes due to brain tumour	15
Pulmonary metastases	21
QUEYRAT's erythroplasia	32
RADIATION, background, and tumour formation	58
— factor in tumour formation	44, 56
— workers in field of, cancer in	57, 63
Radioactive atoms, ionizing alpha- and beta-particles of, causing cancer	57
Radiotherapy	92
Radon inhalation causing lung cancer	57
Rectal polyp	37
Rectum, cancer of, prognostic classification	10
Red blood-cell, ultimate in differentiation	29
Redifferentiation of cells	27
Reduction division of germ cells	101
Regression 38, 40	
Remission in leukaemia in response to drug	39
Renal carcinoma causing polycythaemia	16
— pelvis, tumour of, obstructing ureter	14

	PAGE
Reticulo-endothelial system, affecting immunity	17
— — tumours of	24
— — — chemotherapy for	94, 96
— — — spread of	23, 24
Retinoblastoma	50
Retroperitoneal teratoma	98, 101
— tumour obstructing ureter	13
Rhabdomyoma	7
Ribosenucleic acid (*see* RNA)	
Ring stricture due to colonic cancer	13
RNA	47
— as viral component	70
— viruses, incorporation of, into cell genome	71
Rous sarcoma virus	66
Rubber workers, bladder cancer in	63
SACROCOCCYGEAL teratoma	98, 101
Salivary tumours, mixed (*Fig.* 5)	9, 30
Sarcoma(ta) (*see also under specific parts*)	
— due to plastic film implants	56
— histology of	28
— invading blood-vessels	21
— with rare metastases	5
Schistosomiasis, bladder cancer associated with	56
Scrotal cancer of chimney sweeps	58, 60
Sebaceous adenomata of tuberose sclerosis	17
Seminoma of testis, cellular reaction of host to	87
Sensory function, loss of, due to tumour	15
Serous effusion due to tumour	12
Sex chromatin particle in teratomata	99, 101
— difference in tumour incidence	89
Sexual development, hormones influencing	77
Shope papilloma virus	66
Sickle-cell disease, Burkitt's lymphoma and	52, 69
Simian virus 40	67
Single-gene genetics, classic, tumours associated with	48
Skin cancer due to ultra-violet radiation	56
— — in X-ray workers	57
— carcinoma due to long-continued trauma	56
— diseases and tumour formation	17
— eruptions, non-specific, associated with tumours	17
— metastases	20
Smoking, lung cancer associated with	61
Spinal cord metastases	23
— metastases	22

110

INDEX

Splenic transplants and tumour formation, in animals 82
Squamous carcinoma, disorderly proliferation of cells around .. 34
Squamous-cell carcinoma, differentiation in 29
— — of skin associated with long-continued trauma 56
Stem cells 27
Steroid drugs (see Corticosteroids)
— hormones, excess of 76
Stilboestrol treatment of prostatic cancer 83, 84
Striated-muscle tumours 7
Strontium, radioactive, danger from fall-out of 58
Struma ovarii 10
Sunlight and skin cancer 56
Surgery for tumours, pathological basis of 92
Susceptibility of animal species to different tumours 48
— to tumour development .. 51

Tar as cause of skin cancer 44, 58, 60
Teratocarcinoma 10
Teratoma (see also under specific parts) 9, 78, 79, (Figs. 13–16) 98
— embryology 98
— endocrine activity of 16
— histological appearance of (Figs. 14–16) 99
Testicular teratoma 79
— — sex chromatin in .. 99, 101
— tumours, sexual effects of .. 77
Testis, choriocarcinoma of, remission of primary tumour .. 41
— chorionepithelioma of 9
— hormone secretion by 77
— seminoma of, cellular reaction of host to 87
— teratoma of 98, 101
— — endocrine activity of .. 16
Therapeutic radiation causing cancer 57
— régime, adaptation of tumour cells to 39, 40, 83
Thioguanine, 6- 94, 96
Thorium, therapeutic, causing cancer 57
Thrombophlebitis migrans .. 17
Thyroid cancer due to X-ray therapy to thymus 57
— carcinoma, metastatic, hormone production by .. 73, 74
— — phaeochromocytoma associated with 49
— gland, hormones of 74
— medullary carcinoma of, associated with phaeochromocytoma 80

Thyroid medullary carcinoma producing excess of calcitonin .. 75
— — — prostaglandin level associated with 80
— spinal metastases of 22
— tumour causing hyperthyroidism 74
— — iodine-concentrating, radioactive isotope treatment of 92
Thyrotrophic hormone, tumours producing 81
Tissue transplantation, host versus graft reaction 85
TNM system of classification of tumours 10
Totipotent cell rests as origin of teratoma 100
Toxic effects of tumour 15
Trauma, long-continued, tumour formation associated with .. 55
Trophoblastic tumour transmitted to mother 87
Tuberose sclerosis 30, 32, 50
Tumour(s), aberrant hormone production by 80
— association of, with other genes 52
— causing damage to vital structures 15
— cells, changes in, during progression 38
— — evolution of cell-mediated immunity to combat .. 90
— characteristics 3
— chemotherapy of, pathological basis of 92
— chromosomes and 53
— classification .. (Figs. 2–6) 6
— clinicopathological correlation in 11
— development, susceptibility to .. 51
— differentiation in 28
— distinction between malignant and benign 4, 7
— emboli in blood-vessels 13
— endocrine deficiency due to .. 81
— of endocrine organs, hormone-secreting 16
— formation, environmental factors 55
— and genetics 47
— general effects 15
— histology 28
— hormones and 73
— — as aetiological factors in .. 82
— — in treatment of .. 83, 84
— immunity and 85
— intermediate between benign and malignant .. (Figs. 2–4) 5, 7
— local effects 11
— mass, local effects 11
— necrosis causing perforation of viscus 14
— — infective 14
— origin of (see Oncogenesis)
— reaction of host to 87

III

INDEX

	PAGE
Tumour(s) regression of	40
— spread of	19
— transplantation	86, 87
— undetectable primary	24
— viruses and	65
— — in treatment of	71
Tumour-cell antigens	86
Turner's syndrome, association of gonadal tumours with	54
Twin pregnancy theory of origin of teratoma	100, 101
Two-stage hypothesis of oncogenesis	44, 46
Tylosis	50
ULCERATIVE colitis, colonic cancer associated with	56
Ultra-violet light, abnormal sensitivity to, in xeroderma pigmentosa	51
— radiation causing skin cancer	56
Umbilical cord, teratoma-like mass in	101
Ureteric obstruction due to pelvic tumour	13
Ureters, spread of metastases along	20, 23
Urethane	94, 96
— causing cancer	62
Urethra, prostatic carcinoma obstructing	13
Urinary calculi due to parathyroid tumour	76
Urine, excretion of carcinogenic substances in, causing bladder cancer	63
Uterine cervix (see Cervical; Cervix)	
Uterus, carcinosarcomata of	9, 30
— distortion due to fibroids	14
— fibroid, benignancy of	5
— — enormous	15
— spread of metastases to and from	23
VAGINA, metastases in	23
Vascular obstruction due to tumour	13

	PAGE
Vegetable compounds, antitumour	94, 96
Venereal sarcoma in dogs, transmission	65
Verruca vulgaris, viral oncogenesis of	68
Vinblastine and vincristine	94, 96
Viral genetic material incorporated into cell genome	70, 71
— — — tumour cell genome	71
— infection enhancing immunological potential	71
— multiplication in and destruction of cell	70
— — tumour cell	71
— oncogenesis in animals	65
— — man	68
— — mechanism	70
— tumours, antigenic structure of cells of	86
— — viral component in cells of	70
Virus(es), activation of dormant, and carcinogenesis	59
— 'particles' in blood in leukaemia	69
— passenger	70
— in treatment of tumours	71
— and tumours	65
Visceral obstruction by tumour	13
Von Hippel-Lindau syndrome	49
WART, viral oncogenesis of	68
Wilms's tumour	48
XERODERMA pigmentosa	32, 51, 56
X-ray(s) as cause of cancer	57
— examination in pregnancy, danger of	57
ZINC as carcinogen	62
Zollinger-Ellison syndrome	77, 80
Zuckerkandl, organs of, adrenal tumours of	76